MARKERS OF CHEMICALLY INDUCED CANCER

MARKERS OF
CHEMICALLY INDUCED
CANCER

Edited by

Gustave Freeman

SRI International
Menlo Park, California

and

Harry A. Milman

Office of Toxic Substances
U.S. Environmental Protection Agency
Washington, DC

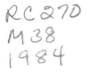

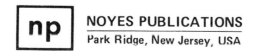

NOYES PUBLICATIONS
Park Ridge, New Jersey, USA

Library of Congress Catalog Card Number: 83-23617
ISBN: 0-8155-0972-3
Printed in the United States

Published in the United States of America by
Noyes Publications
Mill Road, Park Ridge, New Jersey 07656

10 9 8 7 6 5 4 3 2 1

Library of Congress Cataloging in Publication Data

Main entry under title:

Markers of chemically induced cancer.

    Bibliography: p.
    Includes index.
    1. Tumor markers. 2. Cancer- -Diagnosis.
3. Carcinogenesis. 4. Carcinogenicity testing.
I. Freeman, Gustave. II. Milman, Harry A. [DNLM:
1. Carcinogens, Environmental. 2. Neoplasms- -
Chemically induced. 3. Neoplasms- -Diagnosis. QZ
202 M345]
RC270.M38 1984   616.99'4075   83-23617
ISBN 0-8155-0972-3

Preface

The production of chemicals and their distribution in commerce have increased substantially over the last 20 to 30 years. It is estimated that about 1,000 new chemicals enter the environment in significant amounts each year. The ability of some chemicals to induce cancer in exposed populations is of major concern to human health. Currently, the best method to detect carcinogens is the long-term animal bioassay. However, the assay lacks sensitivity, is expensive, resource intensive, and very time consuming. Therefore, methods are needed which can identify carcinogens but are of shorter duration and less costly in order to expedite the process of cancer prevention.

This review focuses on biochemical and immunological changes that correlate with carcinogenicity. Such "markers," if occurring early enough, may be used to predict the onset of cancer in experimental animals exposed to potential chemical carcinogens long before morphological changes are seen. Furthermore, the judicious use of biological markers, along with analysis of structure-activity relationships and results from mutagenicity assays, cell-transformation tests and limited bioassays, may increase (or decrease) the "weight of the evidence" for the carcinogenicity of chemical compounds. It is by examining all the information available about the potential carcinogenicity of chemicals that proper decisions can be made towards limiting the risk of cancer due to exposure to chemical carcinogens.

Menlo Park, California
Washington, DC
July, 1983

Gustave Freeman
Harry A. Milman

v

Acknowledgments

This review was prepared by the staff of the Life Sciences Division of SRI International in collaboration and under contract with the U.S. Environmental Protection Agency (EPA Contract No. 18-01-5079).

We are grateful for the critical reviews and comments offered by Drs. K. Robert McIntire, Stewart Sell, and E.K. Weisburger, members of the Health and Environmental Review Division of the Office of Toxic Substances of the EPA, and Dr. Freddy Homburger.

Without the patient indulgence and dedication of the secretarial and administrative personnel throughout several revisions, this review of a massive literature could not have been realized, and we are grateful to those who have contributed.

Disclaimer

Contributors

The contributors listed below are from SRI International, Menlo Park, California.

L.J. Anderson	Cell Biologist
A.E. Brandt	Senior Biochemist
W.E. Davis	Senior Cancer Biologist
G. Freeman	Director, Department of Medical Sciences
P.Y. Fung	Biochemist
S.J. Gee	Toxicologist
C.T. Helmes	Director, Biological and Environmental Chemistry
R.A. Howd	Senior Biochemical Pharmacologist
H.L. Johnson	Chemist
L.T. Juhos	Director, Inhalation Toxicology
M.J. Lipsett	Senior Policy Analyst
V.J. McGovern	Chemist
E.F. Meierhenry	Director of Pathology
R.M. Miao	Senior Biochemist
J.P. Miller	Director, Biotechnology Research
H.A. Milman*	Pharmacologist
P.A. Papa	Chemist
C.C. Sigman	Director, Chemical-Biological Information
D.G. Streeter	Developmental Cell Biologist
R.H. Suva	Biochemist
C.A. Tyson	Director, Biochemical Toxicology
B.S. Vold	Senior Biochemist
K.J. Westsik	Senior Librarian
A. Winship-Ball	Toxicologist

*Office of Pesticides and Toxic Substances, U.S. Environmental Protection Agency.

Abbreviations

2-AAF	2-Acetylaminofluorene
o-AAT	o-Aminoazotoluene
ACTH	Adrenocorticotropin hormone
ADH	Antidiuretic hormone
AFB_1	Aflatoxin B_1
AFP	Alpha-fetoprotein
AHH	Aryl hydrocarbon hydroxylase
ALL	Acute lymphoblastic leukemia
ALP	Alkaline phosphatase
AP	Acid phosphatase
APUD	Amine precursor uptake and decarboxylation
BA	Benz(a)anthracene
β_2-M	β_2-Microglobulin
BHC	Hexachlorocyclohexane, γ-isomer
BHT	Butylated hydroxytoluene
BP	Benzo(a)pyrene
Ca	Cancer antigen
Ca1	Cancer antibody
C-cells	Calcitonin-producing cells
CEA	Carcinoembryonic antigen
CD	Choline-deficient
CSF	Cerebrospinal fluid
CMP-NANA	Cytosine-5'-monophosphoryl-N-acetylneuraminic acid
CNS	Central nervous system
DAB	4-Dimethylaminoazobenzene
3'-Methyl-DAB	3'-Methyl-4-dimethylaminobenzene
2,4-DAT	2,4-Diaminotoluene
DCMP	Deoxycytidylate

DDT	Dichlorodiphenyltrichloroethane
DEN	Diethylnitrosamine
DES	Diethylstilbestrol
DMAB	Dimethylaminobenzene
DMBA	Dimethylbenzanthracene
DMN	Dimethylnitrosamine
DNA	Deoxyribonucleic acid
DNT	Dinitrotoluene
64DP	A DNA binding protein in serum
EDTA	Ethylenediaminetetraacetic acid
EH	Epoxide hydrolase
FAA	N-2-Fluorenylacetamide
FDP	Fructose diphosphate
FSA	Fetal sulfoglycoprotein antigen
FSH	Follicle-stimulating hormone
GC	Gas chromatography
GDH	Glutamate dehydrogenase
GGT	γ-Glutamyltranspeptidase
GOT	Glutamate oxaloacetate transaminase
G6P	Glucose-6-phosphatase
G6PD	Glucose-6-phosphate dehydrogenase
GPAD	Glycylprolinedipeptidylaminopeptidase
GPN	Glycylpropyl-p-nitronilidase
GPT	Glutamide-pyruvate transaminase
GM_3	N-Acetylneuraminic acid-galactose-glucose-N-acetylsphingosine
GT-II	Serum galactosyltransferase isoenzyme II
HBB	Hexabromobiphenyl
HBB	$3,3',4,4',5,5'$-Hexabromobiphenyl
HCC	Hepatocellular carcinoma
HCG	Human chorionic gonadotropin
HCH	Hexachlorocyclohexane
HPLC	High-performance liquid chromatography
LAP	Leucine aminopeptidase
LDH	Lactate dehydrogenase
LH	Luteinizing hormone
3-MC	3-Methylcholanthrene
2-MeDAB	2-Methyl-4-dimethylaminoazobenzene
$3'$-MeDAB	$3'$-Methyl-4-dimethylaminobenzene
$4'$-MeDAB	$4'$-Methyl-7-dimethylaminoazobenzene
MFO	Mixed function oxidase (monooxygenase)
mg	Milligram
MNNG	N-Methyl-N$'$-nitro-N-nitrosoguanidine
MNU	N-Methyl-N-nitrosourea
MSP	Melanoma-specific protein
MTC	Medullary thyroid cancer
N	Number
NADPH	Nicotinamide adenine dinucleotide phosphate (reduced)

5'-Nase	5'-Nucleotidase
NADH	Nicotinamide adenine dinucleotide (reduced)
N-OH-FAA	N-Hydroxy-N-2-fluorenylacetamide
NNM	N-Nitrosomorpholine
5'-NPDase	5'-Nucleotide phosphodiesterase
α_2-PAG (or α_2-PAM)	Pregnancy-associated α_2-glycoprotein
PAM	Pregnancy-associated macroglobulin
PB	Phenobarbital
PEP	Phosphoenol pyruvate
pg	Picogram
PH	Partial hepatectomy
PLAP	Placental alkaline phosphatase
PRL	Prolactin
PTH	Parathyroid hormone
RBC	Erythrocyte (red blood cell)
RNA	Ribonucleic acid
RNase	Ribonuclease
SDH	Sorbitol dehydrogenase
SMC	Seromucoid
SP_1	Pregnancy-associated glycoprotein$_1$
SP_3	Pregnancy-associated glycoprotein$_3$
TA	Thioacetamide
TCDD	2,3,7,8-Tetrachlorodibenzo-p-dioxin
TDT	Terminal deoxynucleotidyl transferase
TK	Thymidine kinase
TMP	Thymidylate
TPA	Bjorklund's tissue polypeptide antigen
tRNA	Transfer ribonucleic acid
tRNA^{Trp}	Tryptophanyl tRNA
TSH	Thyroid-stimulating hormone
UDP	Uridine diphosphate
ZGM	Zinc glycinate marker

Contents and Subject Index

I

Introduction

G. Freeman

The search for early manifestations of cancer has been a
major preoccupation, especially after surgical excision and
irradiation were shown to be reasonably effective treatments
for the disease. When epidemiologic evidence of cancer
became associated with occupation, as in the historic case
of skin cancer among chimney sweeps, the concept of prevention in the control of cancer became paramount.

The environmental biologist is concerned mainly with prevention, so that tests are sought to distinguish between
exogenous cancer-inducing factors and relatively benign
ones. A putative clue for induction of cancer is termed
a "marker," a term used widely as a synonym for "indicator"
in biologic research (Sell, 1980). During recent decades,
epidemiology has stigmatized X-irradiation and smoking
of tobacco irrevocably as major examples among causative
factors in cancer. Obviously, epidemiology is an essential
and effective exploratory probe, usually after the fact.
Such studies in man are often hampered by time, expense,
and lack of available expertise. Both old and newly introduced chemical, physical, and infectious elements are yet
to be evaluated among the enormous number and kaleidoscopic
varieties that pollute the environment (USPHS, 1981).

The conventional criteria used in the clinic--symptoms,
physical signs, evidence of bleeding, visualization by
various invasive and noninvasive techniques, and histologic
examination of accessible tissues--summarize the main
current technologic armamentarium by which diagnosis of

malignant tumors is achieved. The percentage of curable cases for several types of cancer has been rising as a result of growing public awareness of signs and symptoms, through epidemiology (National Institutes of Health, 1981), and with improvements in diagnosis and therapy. Nevertheless, cancer remains the second most prevalent category of diseases causing death in the United States (National Center for Health Statistics, 1982).

Several comprehensive monographs on cancer markers have been published (Ruddon, 1978; Herberman, 1980; Sell, 1980; Statland, 1981; Sell and Wahren, 1982; Chu, 1982; Busch, 1982). The subject remains diffuse. It presents a circular problem that inadvertently poses basic questions such as, "What precipitates or inaugurates the malignant behavior of cells, and what molecular phenomena determine subsequent oncogenesis?" As these aspects, which are being probed vigorously, become clearer, better markers will be identified. Meanwhile, rather broad associations have been made between the established state of cancer and (1) genetic susceptibility (Marks, 1981) and (2) the reappearance of cellular products usually expressed only in embryonic life (Abelev et al., 1963; Gold and Freedman, 1965; Pearson and Freeman, 1968) and often during the regeneration of injured tissue.

Unless cancer is an inherent condition of life that tends to remain under control through immunologic or other surveillance mechanisms, one must turn to the regulation of genetic expression to look for the "rogue" genes and their regulatory elements that determine oncogenesis (Levinson et al., 1978; Klein, 1981; Bishop, 1981; Bishop, 1982).

The objective of this review is to identify early biochemical events induced by chemicals in the environment that lead experimentally to the development of cancer in animals. Results in experimental animals treated over a relatively short period of time, including oncogenesis, were investigated. The review was limited to recent literature dealing with human subjects as well as animals, because observations and methods that have been proven to be fruitful in one species might apply to another. The great majority of reports are on human cancer, but they often describe studies with animals also (Chu, 1982; Ruddon, 1978; Sell, 1980; Sell and Wahren, 1982; Statland, 1981).

Where does the concept of "marker" fit in the sequential development of cancer? Its contemporary usage is in terms of a biochemical and/or immunologic phenomenon that is significantly, but not uniquely, associated with cancer. The more specific and sensitive the test for cancer (or of a precancerous state), the more effective will be the reduction in the proportions of false-negative and false-positive tests. Thus, the selection of markers useful for prevention and early diagnosis will have been advanced (Statland, 1981).

For this review, we define a marker as an aberration of normal metabolism that is associated with a preneoplastic or an early stage of cancer and can be detected and measured in animals or man. Techniques for detecting several types of cancer have already been established or are being improved in specificity and sensitivity so that a given marker can be shown to be present (1) only in a host developing cancer, or (2) in concentrations that are significantly higher or lower than in the body fluids or tissues of otherwise comparable normal individuals of the same species.

In contrast to the vast number of clinical observations in humans, surprisingly few biochemical or immunologic studies of the preneoplastic state have been applied in animals. Nevertheless, well over 500 chemicals having putative onco-genic influence, as selected by the National Cancer Insti-tute, have been or are being studied in laboratory bioassays (NTP, 1982; USPHS, 1981).

Thus, identifying persons who are either "at high risk" of developing cancer (Marks, 1981) or actually harbor malignant tissue that is amenable to eradication has been a critical issue, assuming that the potential for total prevention or cure of all cancer is not yet on the horizon. An intensive search is under way in laboratories and clinics around the world for biochemical, immunologic, and other tests in man and animals that may reveal evidence of impending or early existence of cancer.

Markers do not constitute a specific biochemical category; they fall into several groups depending on their biochemical structure, origin, physiologic function, and ability to incite specific immunologic or pathologic responses. Thus, the methods of detection may be relatively simple and inex-pensive, or complex and costly. Whether or not a marker or a profile of markers will become useful in screening large populations will depend, in part, on economics. However, a marker may prove to be an invaluable tool with which to

probe mechanisms that may reveal ways of ultimately controlling malignant growth and thereby neutralize "cost-benefit"
as a practical consideration. For obvious reasons, environmental chemicals require testing for putative harmful characteristics in selected animal species or cellular systems.

Specificity for a neoplastic cell type, tissue, or organ
would greatly enhance a marker's value for illuminating
oncogenic mechanisms as well as for revealing the site
clinically. Using the criteria of specificity and sensitivity, efforts have been made to formulate and assign a
numeric value for each putative marker for comparison with
the distribution of each of the two characteristics in a
normal population. Such values, in turn, are compared
statistically with values in equivalent subpopulations suspected of being at risk or of having nononcogenic diseases
(Statland, 1981). Clearly, specificity is paramount, and
sensitivity is subject to improvement.

Laboratory animal models have been used extensively to test
the mutagenicity and oncogenicity of chemicals (and their
mixtures) and of infectious (viral) and physical agents.
Although the dosages used in laboratory experiments almost
always include high levels not likely to be experienced by
man, an impressive correlation exists between the probability of inducing cancer in some organ system or tissue of an
animal and the probability of its occurrence in man exposed
by virtue of his occupation or residence, or iatrogenically
(Tomatis, 1979). Vulnerability to an inducing agent varies
with the animal species, the route and regimen of administration, and the tissue(s) likely to be affected, in addition to the background factors of sex, age, genetic strain,
and indigenous viral infection.

Despite numerous variables that are inherent in both animal
and human investigations of oncogenesis and its early diagnosis (Lokich, 1978), the enormous effort over the past
decades, especially in regard to human cancer, has generated
meaningful data. This has resulted from improved experimental designs, sophistication of epidemiology, genetic
concepts, and the development of new analytic laboratory
techniques. Procedures for screening compounds for putative
oncogenicity in laboratory animals have been standardized
in recent years by the National Cancer Institute and the
National Toxicology Program and are being improved in several laboratories (NTP, 1982). Results from these and
global sources (Tomatis, 1979) were compared and evaluated.

Genetically susceptible humans and animals, subject to exposure to contaminated air, food, water, or topical chemical or physical incitants of neoplasia, may become victims of "initiation" (Farber, 1981) in the sense of the generally accepted concept that cancer proceeds from preliminary contact with such an oncogenic factor and is then "promoted" by a critical second factor (Farber, 1982) that is likely to be reversible and nononcogenic by itself, although indirectly disruptive to DNA. The probability of encountering or harboring an effective promoter, as well as an initiator, may be relatively low but is relevant to large populations. Considering the probable ubiquity of initiators and promoters, the frequency of their interdependence may be exaggerated in certain occupations and industrialized areas. Promotion in experimental animals, however, can be a controllable factor.

To study the basic mechanisms involved in cellular changes that lead to the malignant growth of cells, several model systems have been developed using chemicals, viruses, and physical types of inducers in cell and tissue cultures, in animals, and in their progeny. The genetic susceptibility of animals (including man) and plants for developing malignant growth is readily shown in certain inbred strains of laboratory animals, in which the large majority die of cancer. Other inbred strains of the same species give rise to progeny that die at equivalent or more advanced ages of diseases other than cancer (Marks, 1981).

The concept of earliest biochemical deviations from "normal," having statistical validity, rests uneasily on a bed of variables inherent in the infinite complexity of biology. Genetic variability is critical but can be controlled reasonably well in an animal species by inbreeding or by cloning cells in culture; such lines may be selected to differ from others in terms of response to a particular oncogenic factor. Both high- and low-risk strains of experimental animals within a species have been developed genetically for comparative studies of induced markers. However, only in certain identifiable human families, as in carriers of xeroderma pigmentosum, for example, do phenotypes indicate a high degree of specific susceptibility to cancer (Marks, 1981). Although proneness to cancer among particular HLA types is recognized, for the most part the probability of individual human risk for cancer remains unpredictable, except in statistically controlled groups

associated with identifiable, influential environmental
factors.

Thus, the interdependence between inciting factors and
identification of individuals and populations at risk calls
for specific, sensitive, and relatively rapid and inexpensive methods for their recognition. Various tests for
effects of chemicals are either in use currently or under
development and are based on the mutagenicity of bacteria,
the induction of chromosomal aberrations in eukaryotic cells
in culture and, also, on the use of long-term exposures of
animals. "Prognostic" shorter-term, direct animal assays
for chemical oncogenesis, however, remain a compelling need
(NTP, 1982) and are addressed in this review.

Enzyme activities, proteins, polypeptides such as hormones,
and oncofetal cellular products are measured directly in
samples of body fluids or tissues or are assayed biologically. A powerful but less quantitative method for use
in animals is microscopic cytochemistry, by which changes
in cellular and tissue structure and staining characteristics can be compared over a time course from the putative
induction of oncogenesis to its overt manifestation in
animals (Culling, 1974; ILAR, 1980). This applies to all
organs, tissues and their cells and can include rapidly
developing immunologic radiolabeling and fluorescence
methods even on fixed tissue (Culling, 1974; Taylor, 1981).
Such visible effects may be correlated with selected
biochemical changes (qualitative and quantitative) in
accessible body fluids.

The search for early or preneoplastic stages has revealed
methods that might prove to be specific and sensitive for
detecting an oncogenic process. The successful tracking
of a process would incorporate evidence of preliminary
stages that have progressed to an induced overt neoplasm.
Methods used for this purpose in the whole animal have been
morphologic, biochemical, histochemical, and immunologic.
Immunology has been used to detect novel proteins generated
by the host and released by oncogenic cells into the circulation and to recognize such antigens on the surfaces of
circulating and fixed cells. Antibodies can be complexed
with radiolabeled probes to recognize cancer-associated
circulating elements containing antigenic adducts. They may
be assayed immunologically in blood or urine or on antigen-
containing tissue. Also, tumor-associated antigen-antibody
complexes can be detected. The selectivity and sensitivity

of immunologic methods have been enhanced greatly by the rapidly growing application of monoclonal antibodies derived from hybridomas (Köhler and Milstein, 1975).

Increasingly, attention is being focused on interactions between oncogenic chemicals, physical or viral agents (or their biochemically activated intermediates), and genetic material at the chromosomal (Rowley, 1980), mitochondrial, and molecular levels (Klein, 1981), and how they may alter the regulation of an affected cell's growth. Transpositions, transfection, and epigenetic mechanisms may be invoked when direct point mutations seem improbable but not impossible (Weinberg, 1982).

In reviewing the earliest events that might serve as markers, a major concern is the nature of the target cell. The phenomenon of "spontaneous" oncogenesis in mature animals and man is often allied with elements found in common in embryonic tissue, cancer tissue of related embryologic origin (Gold and Freedman, 1965), and in virally or spontaneously transformed eukaryotic cells in culture (Pearson and Freeman, 1968), but not with mature differentiated normal cells or tissue of the same derivation (Abelev et al., 1963). The most commonplace examples have been CEA (Gold and Freedman, 1965) and AFP (Sell, 1980). This phenomenon is attributed, variously, to failure of repression of a normal growth gene(s), late derepression of such a gene(s), an arrest in differentiation, or an aberration of base modifications (Müller and Rajewsky, 1980).

Another hypothesis for aberrant expression in cell growth implies that eukaryotic cells "normally" contain specific cancer-related genes that may or may not become expressed. However, it is not clear, semantically, whether or not genes that express the products normally required for growth and differentiation are included among those often referred to as "oncogenes." Are "oncogenes" a distinct category with unique sequences (Reddy, 1982), or are they simply expressions of excessive normal gene dosage for growth, determined by translocations or changes in regulatory mechanisms (Bishop, 1981,1982; Cooper, 1980; Klein, 1981; Reddy et al., 1982; Shih et al., 1981; Tabin et al., 1982)?

Some evidence points, also, to kinases that phosphorylate tyrosine or other reacting sites in proteins or peptides, for example. Presumably, such proteins are membrane-bound in the cell. Can such enzymes (or their phosphorylated

reactants) be measured as markers in animal tissues under-
going chemical oncogenesis? Also, do such "new" gene products determine continuous replication of the affected cell
type as well as its stage of differentiation (Twardzik et
al., 1982), or are there several steps in the process of
achieving an irreversible stage?

The ultimate objective would be the detection of such minute
quantities of tell-tale material in body fluids or selected
tissues from experimental animals. Such effective techniques that appear to be too complicated at this time to
serve for screening the oncogenicity of chemicals should
become appropriate methods in time (Logan and Cairns, 1982).
An intensive attack on the problem of determining the direct
or stepwise oncogenicity of chemicals and their mechanisms
of action is likely to evolve into practical means of
identifying impending neoplasia or its eradicable stage.
The use of animals is critical for understanding and then
preventing and controlling chemically induced cancer.

II

Methods

P.A. Papa, C.C. Sigman, L.J. Anderson, K.J. Westsik, V.J. McGovern

A literature search for review articles dealing with "cancer" and "markers" was conducted initially to

- Assess the extent of previous coverage of this subject.

- Obtain key citations for background information.

- Determine the best data bases to be used for data retrieval.

The following on-line data bases (available through Lock-heed's DIALOG® system) were checked for the initial search: MEDLINE, CA SEARCH, EXCERPTA MEDICA, IRL LIFE SCIENCES COLLECTION, and BIOSIS. The results were screened for relevancy, and approximately 220 abstracts were evaluated. MEDLINE and EXCERPTA MEDICA proved to be the most relevant data bases to use for a comprehensive literature search.

The next phase of the literature search focused on the retrieval of information on specific biochemical and immuno-logic markers of cancer from 1975 to the present. A formal literature search was conducted only on markers that appeared to be potential "cancer markers" in terms of an Environmen-tal Protection Agency (EPA) directive; thus, mention of a "marker" in the literature did not necessarily result in the initiation of a search for further information on that marker. At first, searches were made for 21 markers pro-vided by EPA, including ornithine decarboxylase (ODC) and carcinoembryonic antigen (CEA). This list of 21 markers

was expanded to ultimately include 122. These additional
markers were identified from a number of sources:

- Review articles, such as those found in the
  special cancer markers issue of <u>Diagnostic
  Medicine</u> edited by Statland (1981).

- Special books on cancer markers, such as that
  edited by Sell (1980) and several others.

- Abstracts already retrieved during the search
  of the initial 21 markers.

- Current awareness publications such as ISI's
  <u>Current Contents</u>®.

In addition, special searches were conducted when requested
by the staff reviewing the abstracts. For example, several
author searches were done, as well as searches for more
information on "markers" mentioned in such sources as new
articles. Thus, a formal literature search was conducted on
the 122 markers listed in Table II-1, and some information
was sought on other markers (e.g., Clq binding) as requested
by the reviewers. Table II-1 shows that most of the markers
are unique entities (e.g., acid phosphatase), but others
can be categorized as "classes" of markers (e.g., ectopic
hormones, polyamines). Some specific markers (e.g., spermidine) are classified under the broad marker category that
they fall into (e.g., polyamines), but all markers listed
in Table II-1 were specifically included in the literature
search.

The 122 markers were formally searched using MEDLINE from
1975, EXCERPTA MEDICA from 1975, EXCERPTA MEDICA IN PROCESS,
and MEDLINE SDI's (monthly updates of this data base)
through February 1982. To ensure comprehensive coverage of
any particular marker in the data bases, a number of search
terms were used. These included both free-text and thesau-
rus terms (e.g., Medical Subject Headings), common abbrevia-
tions or synonyms, and Enzyme Commission (EC) code (where
appropriate). The search terms identified for each marker
were combined with a variety of truncated cancer terms (e.g,
carcino?, preneopl?, neoplas?, tumo?r?, precancer?) and with
the actual term "marker" (in truncated form). This strategy
provided for the retrieval of information on the use of the
specific biochemical or immunologic marker as it related
to cancer, whether or not the actual term "marker" was used
by the authors. The use of a variety of terms in the initial literature search for each of the markers helped to

eliminate multiple searches for the same marker resulting from the wide variety of names used in the literature to identify a solitary marker. For example, glucanohydrolase is also cited as amylase, glyconase, diastase, ptyalin, and 1,4-α-D-glucan glucanohydrolase (Enzyme Nomenclature, 1978). This approach also allowed material on specific markers, such as pregnancy-specific β1-glycoprotein (SP1), to be retrieved in the same search as material on β-glycoproteins. This helped to provide a means of reviewing related markers together.

The literature search for the 122 markers in both human and animal studies resulted in the retrieval of over 70,000 citations (including numerous citations covering more than one marker) from 1975 through February 1982. Because of the large number of citations and the availability of review articles, books, and other compendia more recent than 1975, only about 2300-2400 citations from 1975-1978 were actually screened and processed. Over 18,000 citations from 1979 through February 1982 were also initially screened for relevancy. From all these citations, approximately 1400 original articles were obtained and formally evaluated by staff reviewers.

The first literature screening was conducted by four investigators. A second screening (of the reduced number of titles and abstracts) was made by 16 reviewers, who selected references that needed to be copied as complete publications. Selected publications were copied by a team making use of the comprehensive Lane Medical Library at Stanford University.

The reviewers, after evaluating a publication (paper or chapter in a book), recorded their critiques on prepared forms, then met in groups organized according to category of "marker" and in keeping with individual interests, experience, and knowledge of the subject.

After group discussions, the individual reviewers prepared written discussions for the elected head of the relevant group, who then organized the material into the appropriate document.

Table II-1

CANCER MARKERS SEARCHED[*]

1. Acetylglucuronidase

2. α_1-Acid glycoproteins

3. Acid phosphatase
   (EC 3.1.3.2)

4. Acute phase proteins

5. 3',5'-Adenosine monophosphate
   (cyclic AMP)

6. S-adenosylmethionine decarboxylase
   (EC 4.1.1.50)

7. Adrenocorticotropic hormone (ACTH)

8. Alcohol dehydrogenase
   (EC 1.1.1.1)

10. Alkaline phosphatase (ALP)
    (EC 3.1.3.1)

11. Aminoacyl-peptide hydrolase
    (leucine aminopeptidase)
    (EC 3.4.11.1)

12. Antidiuretic hormone (ADH; vasopressin)
    arginine vasopressin (AVP)

13. α_1-Antitrypsin (AAT)

14. Aryl amidase

15. Aryl hydrocarbon hydroxylase (AHH)

16. α-Aryl sulfatase
    (EC 3.1.6.1)

---

*Enzyme Commission (EC) numbers and common synonyms are listed where applicable and readily available.

(Continued)

Table II-1 (Continued)

17. Australia antigen

18. Brain-specific antigen (BSA)

19. Branched-chain-amino-acid aminotransferase

20. Breast cyst fluid protein

21. Breast neoplasm chromatin

22. Ca antigen

23. Ca1 antibody

24. Calcitonin

25. Carcinoembryonic antigen (CEA)

26. Carcinofetal ferritins

27. Cathepsin B1
    (EC 3.4.22.1)

28. Ceruloplasmin

29. Chalone factor

30. Colon antigen (not CEA)

31. Contractile proteins

32. Corticotrophin-like-intermediate-polypeptide (CLIP)

33. Creatine kinase
    (EC 2.7.3.2)

34. 3',5'-Cyclic nucleotide phosphodiesterase
    (EC 3.1.4.17)

35. Cystathionine

36. Deoxycytidylate deaminase

(Continued)

Table II-1 (Continued)

37. Diamine oxidase (histaminase)
     (EC 1.4.3.6)

38. DNA nucleotidylexotransferase
     (terminal addition enzyme; terminal
     deoxyribonucleotidyl transferase)
     (EC 2.7.7.31)

39. DNA nucleotidyltransferase (DNA
     polymerase) (EC 2.7.7.7)

40. Ectopic hormones

41. Epoxide hydrolase (EH; epoxide
     hydratase) (EC 3.3.2.3)

42. Erythropoietin

43. Esterases
        blood esterases
        plasma esterases

44. Ferritins

45. Fetal hemoglobin (HBF)

46. Fetal sulfoglycoprotein antigen

47. α-Fetoprotein (AFP)

48. Fibrin-fibrinogen degradation products
     (FDP)

49. Follicle-stimulating hormone (FSH)

50. Fucose

51. α-Fucosidase
     (EC 3.2.1.51)

52. Fucosyl transferase

53. Galactosyl transferase (lactose synthase)
     (EC 2.4.1.22)

(Continued)

Table II-1 (Continued)

54.   Gastric inhibitory polypeptide
       (GIP)

55.   Globulins
         albumin
         immunoglobulins

56.   Glucanohydrolase (amylase)
       (EC 3.2.1.1)

57.   Glucosaminidase
       (EC 3.2.1.30)

58.   Glucose-6-phosphate dehydrogenase
       (EC 1.1.1.49)

59. β-Glucuronidase
       (EC 3.2.1.31)

60.   Glutamate dehydrogenase (GDH)
       (EC 1.4.1.2)

61. γ-Glutamyl transferase (GGT; gamma-
       glutamyltranspeptidase)
       (EC 2.3.2.2)

62. β-Glycoproteins

63.   Glycosidase

64.   Growth hormone (GH)

65.   3',5'-Guanosine monophosphate
       (cyclic GMP)

66.   Hexokinase
       (EC 2.7.1.1)

67.   Hexosaminidase

68.   Human chorionic gonadotropin (HCG)

69.   Human chorionic somatomammotropin (HCS)

70.   Hydroxyproline

(Continued)

Table II-1 (Continued)

71. Insulin

72. Iodine (not thyroid)

73. Isocitrate dehydrogenase
     (EC 1.1.1.41)

74. Isoferritins

75. Lactate dehydrogenase (LDH)
     (EC 1.1.1.27)

76. Lipotropic hormone (LPH)

77. Luteinizing hormone (LH)

78. α-Macrofetoprotein
     (acute phase α_2-macroglobulin)

79. Macrophage electrophoretic mobility assay

80. Malate dehydrogenase
     (EC 1.1.1.37)

81. Mallory bodies

82. Melanocyte stimulating hormone (MSH)

83. Melanoma-specific protein (MSP)

84. β-Microglobulins

85. Mitogenic factor

86. Myelin proteins

87. α-Naphthyl acetate esterase

88. Neurophysin

89. 5'-Nucleotidase
     (EC 3.1.3.5)

90. Neuron-specific enolase

91. Oncomodulin

(Continued)

Table II-1 (Continued)

92. Ornithine decarboxylase (ODC)
     (EC 4.1.1.17)

93. Pancreatic oncofetal antigen

94. Parathormone (parathyroid hormone)

95. Pituitary hormones

96. Placental anemia-inducing factor

97. Placental lactogen (HPL; PL)

98. Polyamines
        spermidine
        putrescine

99. Pregnancy zone protein

100. Prolactin (PRL)

101. Prostatic acid phosphatase

102. Prostatic antigen

103. Protein kinase
     (EC 2.7.1.37)

104. Putative oncofetal antigen

105. Pyruvate kinase
     (EC 2.7.1.40)

106. Retinoic acid binding protein

107. Reverse transcriptase

108. Serum amyloid A protein

109. Sialoglycoprotein

110. Sialyltransferase
     (EC 2.4.99.1)

111. Tennessee antigen

(Continued)

Table II-1 (Concluded)

112. Thrombopoietin

113. Thymidine kinase (TK)
     (EC 2.7.1.21)

114. Thymidine transferase

115. Thymus leukemia antigen

116. Thyroid-stimulating hormone (TSH;
     thyrotropin)

117. Tissue antigens

118. Tumor-associated antigens (TAA)

119. Tumor-specific antigens (TSA)

120. Urine glycoproteins

121. Vasoactive intestinal polypeptide

122. Zinc glycinate

III

Enzymes of Nucleic Acid Metabolism

D.G. Streeter, B.S. Vold

INTRODUCTION

Interference with the synthesis and function of nucleic acids, particularly DNA, is the primary mode of action of virtually every clinically effective anticancer agent used today. The effects of these agents range from interference with the synthesis of early precursors of nucleic acids by antimetabolites such as methotrexate and 5-fluorouracil to interference with the function of DNA itself by alkylating agents such as cyclophosphamide and nitrogen mustard. If changes in nucleic acid metabolism in tumor cells provide useful targets for cancer therapy, it is logical that such changes would also provide indicators of the disease state and perhaps also of a developing neoplastic condition. There are two principal drawbacks to identifying potential markers as readily analyzable indicators of a developing neoplastic condition:

(1) Increases in the enzymes, substrates, and products of nucleic acid biosynthesis are usually associated with rapidly proliferating cells, and are therefore more likely to be associated with growth and repair of normal cells as well as with the malignant state of tumor cells.

(2) The enzymes of nucleic acid metabolism are primarily cell-associated, and changes are therefore not generally measurable as circulating markers or as excreted elements.

With these general restrictions in mind, the potential usefulness of these markers as early indicators of neoplastic
conditions induced by carcinogenic materials is discussed.

DNA SYNTHETIC ENZYMES

DNA Polymerase

Animal Studies: The increased synthesis of DNA in specific
tissues of animals treated with known carcinogens has been
documented in a number of studies and correlates well with
the subsequent establishment of neoplasms. Studies have
been performed in both rats and mice with compounds such
as N-2-fluorenylacetamide, 4-nitroquinoline-1-oxide, methyl-
methane sulfonate, and benzo(a)pyrene (Stewart, 1981). The
majority of these studies deal with changes in DNA synthesis in hepatocarcinogenesis (Stewart, 1981; Norpoth et al.,
1980; Laishes and Rolfe, 1980; Schulte et al., 1981; Chan
and Becker, 1979), although the correlation also extends
to studies on lung (Rasmussen et al., 1981), colon (Lipkin,
1974), and uterine tissues (Kang and West, 1980). The
simplest way to measure this parameter is by measuring
radiolabeled thymidine incorporation into specific tissues,
either by direct liquid-scintillation counting of tissue
samples (Norpoth et al., 1980; Rasmussen et al., 1981) or
by autoradiography of tissue slices (Laishes and Rolfe,
1980; Schulte et al., 1981; Lipkin, 1974; Kang and West,
1980). Either method yields results within 24 to 48 hours
of tissue sampling. Other methods require the more involved
determination of a specific type of DNA synthesis, the
repair of pre-existing DNA as opposed to the synthesis of
new DNA (Stewart, 1981; Rasmussen et al., 1981), or the
isolation and quantitation of specific DNA polymerases (Chan
and Becker, 1979). This enzyme activity therefore is a
good potential early neoplastic marker in animals because
of the clear association of changes in this activity with
the establishment of precancerous conditions in animals
induced by known carcinogens, and the availability of relatively simple methods to measure it. These factors may
offset the deficiency of requiring a tissue evaluation.

Clinical Studies: Limited clinical studies have also demonstrated increased DNA synthesis and DNA polymerase activity
associated with the transformation of colonic epithelial
cells leading to colon cancer (Lipkin, 1974) and with human
primary hepatomas compared to normal liver (Cummins and

Balinsky, 1980). However, Cummins and Balinsky (1980) found that the increase in DNA polymerase activity associated with human hepatomas was small in comparison with that in the corresponding rat hepatoma. A distinct DNA polymerase activity (DNA polymerase Cm) has also been found in a human melanoma cell line (Loewenstein et al., 1980). The enzyme was not detected in various normal tissues and was found in seven of 14 (50%) malignant tissues examined.

Besides the limited data associating this marker with early neoplastic conditions, there is no information on its induction by chemical carcinogens. Nevertheless, the ubiquitous presence and function of this enzyme activity in both animals and humans suggest that the animal evaluations discussed above may be applicable to predicting the effects of carcinogens in man.

Terminal Deoxynucleotidyl Transferase (TDT)

TDT is an unusual enzyme having an activity related to DNA polymerase that is normally found only in thymus tissue. High levels of activity have been found in certain leukemia cells, and TDT is therefore a potential circulating marker for detecting the presence of that neoplastic condition.

Animal Studies: TDT is readily detectable in leukemic T-lymphocytes induced in mice either by radiation (Bumol et al., 1980) or viruses (Pepersack et al., 1980). Pepersack et al. (1980) found that the TDT positive leukemic cells constitute only one third of the leukemic cell population and are primarily of thymic origin.

The enzyme activity can be determined by a simple radiolabeling assay or by radioimmunoassay and immunofluorescence (Pepersack et al., 1980). A comparison of the enzymes from the peripheral blood lymphocytes of the gibbon and of man, both with acute lymphoblastic leukemia (ALL) (Sarin et al., 1980), is an example of the utility of a marker common to animals and man for the diagnosis of this disease. Because this marker is presently limited to ALL, studies must be conducted in animals to ascertain whether known carcinogens induce TDT in peripheral blood lymphocytes before leukemia appears, to determine the predictive value of this marker.

Clinical Studies: The principal value of this marker lies in the numerous clinical studies linking TDT in circulating leukocytes with ALL (McCaffrey et al., 1981; Sarin et

al., 1980; Bollum, 1979; Habeshaw et al., 1979; Vezzoni et
al., 1981; Kalwinsky et al., 1981; Srivastava et al., 1980;
Hutter et al., 1978; Sakamoto et al., 1979; Murphy, 1978).
These reports and others (Janossy et al., 1980; Okamura et
al., 1980; Long et al., 1979; Pangalis and Bentler, 1979;
Coleman et al., 1976) demonstrate that TDT has little or
no association with other forms of leukemia. There are no
clinical data demonstrating that this marker can be induced
by known carcinogenic agents.

In humans, TDT can be readily measured by a variety of techniques including radioimmunoassay (McCaffrey et al., 1981),
immunofluorescence (McCaffrey et al., 1981; Bradstock et
al., 1981; Stass et al., 1979), antibody-linked peroxidase
assay (Jager, 1981), and microenzyme assay (Modak et al.,
1980).

In summary, the well-documented association of TDT with ALL
in both animals and man, and the easy assay of this circulating marker may make TDT a worthwhile marker to pursue in
animal studies designed to determine if TDT can be induced
by known carcinogens and if such induction is associated
with the development of leukemia. These factors may over-
ride the apparently narrow specificity of the marker.

Thymidine Kinase (TK)

Thymidine kinase (TK) in animals is an important enzyme
for the salvage of thymidine to form nucleotides during
increased DNA synthesis in proliferating cells. Increased
TK activity is found in transplantable rat hepatomas induced
by 3'-methyl-4-dimethylaminoazobenzene (Cummins and Balinsky, 1980), in rat submaxillary gland tumors (Herzfeld and
Raper, 1976), and in rat hepatocarcinogenesis induced by
dimethylnitrosamine (Curtin and Snell, 1980). The study
by Curtin and Snell (1980) is most significant because
increased enzyme activity was detectable two weeks after
treatment, well before the initial appearance of preneoplastic nodules at 11 weeks, indicating that the marker is an
early indicator of hepatocarcinogenesis in the rat. Enzyme
activity was measured only in the affected tissues. It
is assayed readily by simple radioisotope incorporation.

Clinical studies have revealed increased TK activity in
colonic cancer (Herzfeld and Greengard, 1980) and some human
malignant lymphomas (Ellins et al., 1981) when compared
to nonneoplastic controls. However, no changes were found

when some primary hepatomas were compared to normal livers (Cummins and Balinsky, 1980), and increased TK activity was associated with nonneoplastic diseases such as herpes virus infection (Salser and Balis, 1976). Elevated TK activity in normal liver tissue from patients with remote (nonhepatic) neoplasms indicates that such activity may not be confined to the affected tissue. It would be worthwhile, therefore, to determine if the increased TK activity associated with hepatocarcinogenesis in rats (Curtin and Snell, 1980) is detectable in circulating peripheral blood lymphocytes, so that it can be readily measured as a circulating marker.

Thymidylate (TMP) Synthetase

Thymidylate (TMP) synthetase is complementary to thymidine kinase as a potential tumor marker because it is important in the de novo (as opposed to salvage) biosynthesis of thymidine nucleotides for DNA synthesis in proliferating cells.

The potential usefulness of this enzyme as a tumor marker in animals lies in its increased activity in rat hepatomas, together with that of TK (Cummins and Balinsky, 1980), and in colonic adenocarcinomas (Wolberg and Morin, 1981). However, a comparative study of TK and TMP synthetase activities in various rat tumors indicated that the latter is less reliable as a tumor indicator (Herzfeld and Raper, 1976). Also, there are no data demonstrating that elevated TMP synthetase activity is an early indicator of neoplasia.

TMP synthetase is important in tumor biology because inhibition of this enzyme is primarily responsible for the therapeutic effect of the antitumor agents 5-flurouracil and methotrexate in man.

Deoxycytidylate Deaminase

Deoxycytidylate (DCMP) deaminase is another enzyme of DNA metabolism that is elevated in rat and human hepatomas (Cummins and Balinsky, 1980). It is, therefore, a potential marker in conjunction with the previously discussed enzymes TK, TMP kinase, TMP synthetase, and DNA polymerase. The increased activity of this enzyme in macroscopically unchanged liver tissue during hepatocarcinogenesis induced in rats by 3'-methyl-4-dimethyl-aminoazobenzene (Simiskova et al., 1980) is particularly significant. Like the other enzymes discussed, DCMP deaminase is readily measured by simple radioisotope incorporation methods.

In summary, at least three of the five enzymes of DNA synthesis discussed above (DNA polymerase, TK, and DCMP deaminase) become elevated in certain tissues as a result of carcinogenic induction before the establishment of neoplasia. Therefore they are potential tissue markers for predicting its development. In addition, elevated levels of TK arising from tumor induction are not necessarily confined to the affected tissue and raise the possibility that these markers are detectable in circulating cells (lymphocytes), which would eliminate the requirement for sampling solid tissue.

Serum Ribonuclease

Ribonuclease, RNase, is the common name for a group of enzymes that degrade ribonucleic acids. Elevated levels of RNase activity have been observed in animals with cancer (Drake et al., 1975; Maor and Mardiney, 1978) as well as in human diseases such as prostatic (Chu et al., 1980), ovarian (Watring et al., 1979; Sheid et al., 1977; Dobryszycka et al., 1979) and pancreatic (Reddi and Holland, 1976; Moossa and Levin, 1981; Holyoke et al., 1979) cancer.

Although most studies have been concerned with human disease, animals have also been studied, and elevated levels of serum RNase have been reported in mice and rats (Maor and Mardiney, 1978). The RNase data from animals showed that as a marker it has high sensitivity but low specificity because high serum levels of RNase occur in diseases of the kidney (Maor and Mardiney, 1978). An interesting study revealed elevated RNase activity in cell-free thymus homogenates from five strains of mice genetically predisposed to leukemia or reticulum cell neoplasms (Drake et al., 1975); increased activity was detectable well before the onset of neoplastic transformation.

In humans, in which early detection is critical, the assay for RNase has proven useful in the diagnosis of malignancies. In ovarian cancer, levels of serum RNase have been used to differentiate malignant from benign growths (Watring et al., 1979). High values have been found to return to normal in 21 of 22 patients following satisfactory response to treatment (Sheid et al., 1977). A combination of RNase and alanyl amino transferase proved to be the most effective marker system when 11 enzymes were studied (Dobryszycka et al., 1979).

Serum RNase has been used also in studies of pancreatic cancer. For example, Reddi and Holland (1976) found serum RNase activity elevated in 90% of pancreatic cancer patients and normal in 90% of patients with other cancers. However, other authors have published less encouraging results, having found serum alkaline phosphatase or fasting serum glucose to be more useful in the diagnosis of early pancreatic cancer (Moossa and Levin, 1981).

The in vitro system for assaying RNase is not technically difficult, but three aspects of the assay need further improvement:

(1)   The manner in which samples are collected and how soon they are assayed may be critical. Sheid et al. (1977) found that it was necessary to exclude leukocytes from the blood samples by a Ficoll-gradient technique to obtain valid results, and that enzyme activity needed to be measured within 24 hours of receiving the blood sample because RNase activity decreases after 48 hours of storage. This problem may be eliminated by careful planning of the assay.

(2)   There is more than one type of RNase. Although initial studies may have treated RNase activity as being due to one type of enzyme, recent investigations have found serum RNase activity in both mice (Drake et al., 1975) and humans (Chu et al., 1979) to be due to at least two different enzyme systems. Identification and purification of RNase could lead to better detection systems, such as the solid-phase fluorescent immunoassay developed for prostatic acid phosphatase in humans (Chu et al., 1979). Particularly promising in this regard is the report of an RIA specific for pancreatic RNase (Weickmann and Glitz, 1982).

(3)   High RNase activity has been observed in nonmalignant disease. A difficulty that cannot be eliminated is the high plasma or serum RNase levels associated with nonneoplastic diseases involving severe hepatic and/or renal failure (Sheid et al., 1977). However, this may be less critical for an animal system to detect carcinogenicity, because initial RNase serum levels could be used to identify a high-risk population, which could then be examined for kidney damage or other irrelevant or contributory disease.

MODIFYING ENZYMES THAT METHYLATE TRANSFER RNA (tRNA)

Transfer RNAs have the highest degree of modified nucleosides of any type of nucleic acid. The most common class
of modified nucleosides results from the addition of methyl
group(s) formed after transcription of the tRNA by a variety
of very specific methylating enzymes termed tRNA methyltransferases (Kerr and Borek, 1972). Inhibitors of the
tRNA methyltransferases can also be present in cells and
affect the activity of these enzymes. The activities of
methyltransferases are also influenced by the presence of
certain inorganic salts and polyamines (Leboy and Glick,
1976), and there are a number of different tRNA methyltransferases, each specific for a different nucleoside modification and/or site on the tRNA. All of these parameters make
the assay of methyltransferases quite complex.

Although the majority of changes reported in tRNAs during
neoplasia have resulted from a deficiency in a specific
modification (Randerath et al., 1981), increases in tRNA
methyltransferases are characteristic of many malignant
tumors, particularly in liver (Balis et al., 1978). Most
of the work with methyltransferases has been done on rats
stimulated with carcinogens. A published sensitive assay
for carcinogen-induced early changes in tRNA methyltransferase activity detected selective changes in liver tRNA
methyltransferases a few days after treatment with acetyl-
aminofluorene or ethionine (Wainfan et al., 1977; Wainfan
et al., 1979). Guanine methylated in the N^2-position is
the principal modification site. Elevated levels of methyltransferases have also been observed in rats treated with
a single dose of promoter; the time course of the enzyme
changes was similar to that for histologically apparent
damage, but the changes could be detected earlier and they
persisted longer after treatment (Wainfan et al., 1981).

Because the assays require a tissue sample, few clinical
studies have been done comparing data from a number of
patients. Nevertheless, tRNA-methylating enzymes from 20
benign tumors of the human ovary were found to be normal
(Sheid et al., 1974), while malignant tumor tissues showed
elevated methyltransferase levels lending supports to the
idea that elevated levels of methyltransferases are a universal attribute of human malignant tissues (Borek, 1980).

Although the studies with methyltransferases have the disadvantages of being complicated, and require a significant

sample of tissue for assays, studies with animals have indicated that elevated levels of methyltransferases may be a very early marker for cancer. Future research concentrating on assay improvement may lead to a simpler assay.

MARKERS IN NEED OF FURTHER STUDY

Reverse Transcriptase

Reverse transcriptase is an RNA-directed DNA polymerase, in contrast to the usual DNA-directed RNA polymerases that occur in all cells. Reverse transcriptase is found in RNA viruses that must have their RNA copied into DNA for their replication and survival. Interestingly, specific tRNAs function as primers for the initiation of DNA synthesis by the viral RNA-directed DNA polymerase. For example, in the avian sarcoma virus, the primer is a tryptophan tRNA. In tumors caused by RNA viruses, the measurement of reverse transcriptase provides a selective marker. However, inherent methodologic difficulties make clinical application impractical now (see Seidenfeld and Marton, 1979).

5'-Nucleotidase

No definitive studies have been reported that link 5'-nucleotidase levels to any neoplastic conditions in animals, and attempts to induce changes in the enzyme levels in animals with liver carcinogens have produced variable or negative results (Lipsky et al., 1981; Renaud et al., 1980; Agostini et al., 1980).

5'-Nucleotidase is readily assayed in serum, and elevation of its serum level is one of the earliest indicators of liver metastases in humans, with a predictive value of about 85% (Coombes et al., 1978; Beck et al., 1978; Korsten et al., 1974; Schwartz, 1978; Kim et al., 1977). However, the correlation of changes in the serum level of 5'-nucleotidase with other forms of cancer is variable or nonexistent (Sheinina and Kutivadye, 1980; Chatterjee et al., 1981; Dao et al., 1980; Catovsky et al., 1981; Laurent et al., 1977; Roberts et al., 1978).

5'-Nucleotide Phosphodiesterase (5'-NPDase)

There are no reports of studies of this marker in animal models.

5'-NPDase, like 5'-nucleotidase, can be readily assayed in
serum, and an abnormal isozyme (5'-NPD-V) is highly predictive of liver metastases in humans (88 to 98% positive correlation) (Pollock et al., 1979; Tsou and Lo, 1980; Mullen
et al., 1976; Tsou et al., 1980). However, the presence of
this marker also correlated with clinically active hepatitis B infection (43%) and with antigen-positive individuals
(14 to 17%) (Lei-Injo et al., 1980). It would, therefore,
appear to be useful only for detecting liver metastases and
their response to clinical therapy, but not as an early predictive indicator of cancer.

Adenosine Deaminase (ADA)

A few clinical studies (Sakamoto et al., 1979; Murphy, 1978;
Janossy et al., 1980) have established that there is a definite increase in circulating levels of adenosine deaminase
associated specifically with the T-lymphocytes of patients
with ALL that is not found in normal T-lymphocytes or non-T-
non-B leukemic lymphoblasts. It may therefore have some
utility as a marker in conjunction with TDT. However, as
with TDT, the absence of human or animal studies regarding
the value of ADA as a preneoplastic indicator severely
limits its current value as a potential marker.

A number of enzymes with insufficient or negative data
relating to their potential as early neoplastic markers in
suitable animal models are listed in Table III-1 along with
their principal deficiencies.

Table III-1

MARKERS OF NO APPARENT UTILITY

Marker	Deficiency	Reference(s)
Adenylate kinase	Insufficient data; narrow tumor specificity	Ronquist et al., 1977; Seidenfeld and Marton, 1979
Alkaline phosphatase	Insufficient data	Sheinina and Kutivadye, 1980
Alkaline phospho-diesterase	Insufficient data	Renaud et al., 1980
Creatine kinase	Insufficient data; poor tumor specificity	De Luca et al., 1981
Creatinine phospho-kinase	Limited tumor specificity; poor sensitivity	Seidenfeld and Marton, 1979; Catalona and Menon, 1981; Wasserstrom et al., 1981
Phosphodiesterase	Insufficient data	Bender, 1979
Phosphoserine phosphatase	Insufficient data	Herzfeld and Greengard, 1980

(Continued)

Table III-1 (Concluded)

Marker	Deficiency	Reference(s)
Protein kinase	Limited tumor specificity; difficult assay	Clawson et al., 1980; Sharma et al., 1980
Purine nucleoside phosphorylase	Limited tumor specificity; insufficient data	Reaman et al., 1981
Pyrophosphatase	Nonspecific	Shatton et al., 1981
Ribose-5-phosphate isomerase	Insufficient data	Mitsuyama, 1979
Thymidylate kinase	Insufficient data	Cummins and Balinsky, 1980

IV

Modified Nucleosides of Ribonucleic Acids

B.S. Vold

INTRODUCTION

Ribonucleic acids (RNAs), particularly transfer ribonucleic
acids (tRNAs), contain a variety of modified nucleosides
that are formed after transcription of the macromolecule
(Hall, 1971). When these RNAs are degraded, the majority
of modified nucleosides do not appear to be catabolized
to any extent in animals or humans and are excreted in
significant amounts in urine (Borek and Kerr, 1972; Chheda,
1970; Nishimura and Kuchino, 1979). Because tRNAs are the
most highly modified class of RNAs, it has been assumed
that turnover of tRNA is the source of excreted modified
nucleosides (Fink and Adams, 1968; Mandel et al., 1966).
Heterogeneous turnover rates of tRNA have been observed
in mammalian cells (Litt, 1975), and evidence for intracellular scavenging of tRNAs with structural abnormality
has been observed (Nomura, 1974). Therefore, it is possible that incorrectly modified tRNAs, which may arise as
part of a neoplastic process, have a much higher turnover
rate than normally modified tRNAs. Whatever their exact
origin, the level of excretion and pattern of certain modified nucleosides in urine have been correlated with the
metabolic or disease state of the individual (see, for
example, the review by Borek, 1980). Speer et al. (1979)
recently reported that the levels of pseudouridine and
N^2,N^2-dimethylguanosine in human urine, evaluated by high-
performance liquid chromatography, could be correlated
with the disease stage, making them potential markers in
the early diagnosis of cancer.

Because of the interest in modified nucleosides as cancer markers, analysis of the levels of nucleosides in urine has been pursued for several years. Although the initial analytic methods using paper or thin-layer chromatography were laborious and not very sensitive, more recent techniques including ion-exchange chromatography, gas-liquid chromatography, and high-performance liquid chromatography (HPLC) have improved the separation and the sensitivity [see reviews by Davis et al. (1979) and Brown et al. (1980)]. The reverse-phase HPLC system for the separation and quantitation of nucleosides in biologic fluids is a rapid, sensitive, and reliable method for the determination of nanogram amounts of ribonucleosides.

Research on the levels of nucleosides found in urine and their variations in cancer has been conducted with both human and animal systems. Although the general phenomenon is the same, each will be discussed separately.

Increased Excretion of Modified Nucleosides in the Urine of Tumor-Bearing Animals

Although many of the studies on the excretion of nucleosides in urine have been done on humans, a number of good studies have used rats and mice. Harada et al. (1973) reported that the excretion of pseudouridine in the urine of rats tripled 35 days after the implantation of Morris hepatoma 7794A. Rats with Novikoff hepatomas were observed to excrete increased levels of 7-methylguanosine (Nishimura and Kuchino, 1979). Elevated excretion of pseudouridine and deoxycytidine was observed in rats bearing Yoshida ascites sarcoma (Shimizu and Fujimura, 1978) and elevated pseudouridine levels were observed in mice with L1210 cancer or with Friend virus leukemia (Nishimura and Kuchino, 1979).

The most encouraging experiments with animals resulted from a study by Thomale and Nass (1982) who followed the urinary excretion rates of 12 modified nucleosides and bases in mice after tumor induction with a single dose of 3-methylcholanthrene. In their system, elevated urinary levels of modified nucleosides and bases could be detected by HPLC before tumors were diagnosable. In addition, mice that received the carcinogen but developed no tumors, as well as the untreated control mice, showed no alteration in the excretion of any of the modified nucleosides and bases (Thomale and Nass, 1982).

Increased Excretion of Modified Nucleosides in the Urine of Cancer Patients

Elevated levels of nucleosides in human urine have been studied by various biochemical techniques, and most recently by HPLC, to find a system useful for early cancer detection or diagnosis (Waalkes et al., 1975). Table IV-1 lists some of the nucleosides that have been studied and showed elevated levels in patients with particular diseases. Excretion of N^2,N^2-dimethylguanosine in patients with Burkitt's lymphoma or leukemia fell to normal during a period of effective chemotherapy and rose again in one subject during relapse, indicating favorable prospects for early detection with this marker (Borek, 1980). It is similarly encouraging that increased levels of urinary excretion of N^2,N^2-dimethylguanosine were detectable as early as stage I and could be correlated with the stage of disease (Speer et al., 1979).

Increased Levels of Modified Nucleosides in the Serum of Cancer Patients

Most of the work on the levels of modified nucleosides in biological fluids has been done with urine, but their levels in serum have been measured by HPLC (Krstulovic et al., 1979; Brown et al., 1980) and by radioimmunoassay (Levine et al., 1975). These studies have indicated levels of certain modified nucleosides to be elevated in cancer patients, but few studies have been done with serum.

OTHER CLASSES OF RNA

Changes in the synthesis of nuclear RNA (Winicov, 1981) and messenger RNA (Atryzek et al., 1980) have been measured in rats treated with a carcinogen, but the complexity of the assay and the requirement for purified cellular components make these less desirable detection systems.

Modified Nucleosides of Deoxyribonucleic Acid (DNA) Induced by Carcinogens

Carcinogens that can act as alkylating agents are known to cause alterations in DNA. Although normal and tumor cells can repair lesions in DNA induced by alkylating agents, certain cell types can repair the damage faster than others (Lerman et al., 1974). Therefore, it might be possible to select cells from a tissue type in which

Table IV-1

TYPES OF PATIENTS SHOWING ELEVATED EXCRETION
OF MODIFIED NUCLEOSIDES

Modified Nucleoside (or base)	Disease	Reference
Methylated purines	Polycythemia vera Acute gouty arthritis	Weissman et al., 1957
Pseudouridine	Leukemia	Adams et al., 1960
Pseudouridine, 1-Methylinosine N^2,N^2-Dimethylguanosine	Lung cancer Leukemia Burkitt's lymphoma Melanoma Ovarian cancer	Mrochek et al., 1974
Pseudouridine	Gout Psoriasis Leukemia Heterozygous oroticaciduria	Adams et al., 1962
N^2,N^2-Dimethylguanosine Pseudouridine	Metastatic breast cancer	Speer et al., 1979

(Continued)

Table IV-1 (Concluded)

Modified Nucleoside (or base)	Disease	Reference
1-Methylinosine N^2,N^2-Dimethylguanosine Pseudouridine 2-Methylguanosine 1-Methyladenosine	Colon cancer	Gehrke et al., 1978
Pseudouridine 1-Methylguanosine 7-Methylguanosine 8-OH-7-methylguanosine	Hodgkins disease	Cooper et al., 1977
N^2,N^2-Dimethylguanosine 1-Methylinosine Pseudouridines	Bronchogenic carcinoma	Coombes et al., 1978
N^2,N^2-Dimethylguanosine Pseudouridine 1-Methylinosine	Breast cancer	Tormey and Waalkes, 1976
N^2,N^2-Dimethylguanosine 1-Methylinosine Pseudouridine	Bladder cancer	Irving, 1977

repair is relatively slow in order to analyze for abnormal nucleosides produced by the carcinogen. The existence of antibodies specific for carcinogen-DNA adducts provides valuable tools for the detection of carcinogen-induced damage in DNA (Poirier, 1981).

Müller and Rajewsky (1980) have established three immunologic methods to quantitate the O^6-ethyldeoxyguanosine produced in the DNA of rats treated with N-ethyl-N-nitrosourea. They have developed an extremely sensitive radioimmunoassay which can quantitate as little as 0.05 pmol of O^6-ethylguanosine. This would allow quantification from hydrolysates of about 100 μg of ethylated DNA. The O^6-ethylguanosine residues are removed rapidly from the DNA of the liver and other tissues by an enzymatic process, although these residues persist in the rat brain DNA.

The problems of selecting the appropriate time to take samples and the necessity of obtaining DNA from the appropriate tissue do not favor this method as a screening technique at present, except in the case of animal studies using a continuous feeding regimen. However, methodology refinement, such as studies on the kinetics of elimination and/or persistence of the modified residues, might make investigation of such modified nucleosides of DNA more practical.

CONCLUSION

Determining urinary levels of modified nucleosides promises to be serviceable as an indicator of early neoplastic changes in both animals and man. HPLC is now the best technique for determining levels of modified nucleosides. A major limitation is that it requires a chromatographic step on an affinity column and an HPLC system operated by a well-trained person. It does have the advantage of quantitating several nucleosides at the same time. Because some nucleosides seem to be better markers than others, it would be desirable to include a broader spectrum of modified nucleosides for such studies. It will be essential, in both animal and human systems, to compare elevations in urinary nucleosides with any that occur in nonneoplastic diseases.

It would also be desirable to gather more data on the serum levels of nucleosides, and investigate the possibility of establishing an immunologic assay for both serum and urine to complement the HPLC techniques.

V

Hepatic and Renal Enzymes: Indicators of Preneoplastic or Early Neoplastic Lesions

C.A. Tyson, S.J. Gee, E.F. Meierhenry

ENZYME MARKERS FOR LIVER AND KIDNEY CARCINOGENESIS

The liver and kidney are the most common target organs for lesions in animal toxicity studies using environmental chemicals (NAS, 1977; Kluwe, 1981). This review focuses on markers that have been used commonly to detect or define hepatic and renal injury and their suitability or promise for early indication of carcinogenicity. None of the indicators reviewed are exclusively toxic to either organ alone, so their value for the detection of hyperplasia in other tissues is also reviewed here. Many indicators in serum are convenient and inexpensive to monitor; membrane-bound indicators are also covered because the frequency of chemically induced tumorigenicity in the liver may justify limited cytochemical examination to supplement serum analysis and so increase sensitivity. These approaches are particularly useful in animal screens that rely on the identification of putative preneoplastic lesions.

Gamma-Glutamyltranspeptidase

Background: Gamma-glutamyltranspeptidase (GGT) is a membrane-bound enzyme that catalyzes the transfer of the γ-glutamyl moiety of glutathione to an amino acid (or peptide) receptor. Its physiologic roles appear to be the transport of extracellular amino acids into cells and the regulation of intracellular glutathione levels (Heinle et al., 1977; Meister, 1976). The enzyme is widely distributed in mammalian tissues, being highest in epithelia of the proximal renal tubules, choroid plexus, jejunal villi, and some other tissues.

The kidney is an excellent source of the enzyme for detailed biochemical studies (Tate et al., 1976; Meister, 1976). In normal liver, GGT is present in the periportal canaliculi of man and dog, but its activity in the bile duct epithelium in rats is low or negligible (Hagerstrand, 1973). In the fetal liver, GGT activity is actually higher than in the kidney, but activity drops off rapidly at birth and continues to decline as the animals mature (Braun et al., 1977). Liver GGT content also increases during aging, gradually reappearing in rats from 30 weeks on (Kitagawa et al., 1980a), with altered GGT-positive foci apparent by 18 months in some strains (Ogawa et al., 1981).

GGT is present in hyperplastic nodules and in rat hepatomas (Fiala and Reuber, 1970; Fiala and Fiala, 1973; Tsuchida et al., 1979; de Gerlache et al., 1980). The enzyme is variously described as having properties very similar to those of the fetal rat liver enzyme in some studies (Taniguchi et al., 1975; Harada et al., 1976; Selvaraj et al., 1981) and to those of the adult rat kidney enzyme in others (Taniguchi et al., 1974; Tsuchida et al., 1979).

Animal Studies: Fiala and Fiala (1973) were the first to show that GGT was a putative early marker for carcinogenesis. They fed various carcinogens (3'-MeDAB, 2-AAF, TA, DL-ethionine, or DMN) in the diet or drinking water to rats for up to 110 days. Histochemical analysis showed that 3'-MeDAB and 2-AAF produced increased GGT activity in the liver during the first week of the regimen. The activity peaked 35 to 63 days later and leveled off thereafter. After 110 days of continuous feeding of the carcinogens, the activity remained high in the livers after discontinuation of the diet. These results suggested that the elevations in GGT were related to the carcinogenic process induced by the chemicals. A single large dose of either of the strong hepatocarcinogens (3'-MeDAB and 2-AAF) given to rats also caused significantly higher GGT levels in livers within 24 to 48 hours [also confirmed in a follow-up study (Fiala et al., 1976)]. TA and DL-ethionine, weak carcinogens, produced slight GGT elevations; a longer induction period was required. The noncarcinogen 2-MeDAB produced only a transient change in liver GGT. Although no groups were carried long enough for overt carcinomas to have developed, the dose levels administered were those known to be capable of producing hepatomas.

Taniguchi et al. (1974) fed rats diets containing either DMAB or 4'-MeDAB (described as a weaker carcinogen) and observed early elevation (within three days) of GGT activity in the liver. With continued feeding, the activity decreased to baseline after 40 days but then became elevated again, eventually reaching levels 40 times higher than normal in the hepatomas produced by DMAB after 140 days, when the study was terminated. No tumors developed with 4'-MeDAB, possibly because the time allowed for tumor formation was too short. Kojima et al. (1981) reported similar biphasic changes in liver GGT activity with rats fed diets containing other carcinogens (3'-MeDAB, DEN or o-AAT).

Boyd et al. (1981) fed rats a semipurified diet containing BP for 6 or 13 weeks. At the 1000 ppm level (but at no lower level), GGT-positive foci were found in the livers at six weeks, the point of sacrifice, and AFP was elevated in the serum. The authors interpreted these signs as evidence for hepatic neoplasia, but noted that BP was not known to be hepatocarcinogenic without the aid of a promoter. AFP, however, is similarly increased with BP at the 100-ppm-level plus 0.05% dietary PB. The composition of the diet also affects hepatocarcinogenesis (e.g., a choline or protein deficiency) and may underlie differences in results and influence the validity of extrapolations in risk assessment for target organs (Hayes and Campbell, 1980).

Kojima et al. (1980b,c) measured both serum and tissue levels of GGT and the enzyme GPAD in rats fed a diet containing 3'-MeDAB. GGT was increased 20-fold in the serum and 50-fold in liver tissue—much more dramatic changes than occurred with GPAD—when carcinomas were clearly recognizable (after the 16th week of feeding). Although less sensitive, the GPAD changes were detectable much earlier in serum (after four weeks) than those of GGT (after 16 weeks but before the detection of hepatomas), and the cytosolic fraction activity of the former was increased, unlike that of GGT, in hepatic cancer tissue at the expense of microsomal enzyme content (Kojima et al., 1980b).

Several investigators carried out more extended histochemical investigations in conjunction with GGT staining to demonstrate that changes in the enzyme's activity were associated with the emergence and proliferation of hyperplastic cell populations or areas in the liver. Kalengayi et al. (1975) obtained histochemical evidence of strong GGT activity in cell membranes and cytoplasms of rats given AFB_1 for 10 weeks by gastric intubation, concurrent with the appearance of hyperplastic liver foci. These changes were observed after 15 weeks and progressively increased in number and size up to 44 weeks, by which time well-differentiated hepatocellular tumors and carcinomas had developed.

Kuhlmann et al. (1981) gave NNM in drinking water to female Lewis rats for 64 to 250 days and found that GGT was elevated in liver hyperplastic nodules by 94 days and remained elevated after discontinuation of the NNM treatment until the animals were sacrificed (from 2 to 25 weeks later), by which time liver tumors had developed. Boelsterli and Zbinden (1979) earlier gave NNM in drinking water at about the same intake level to male rats and used repeated fine-needle aspiration biopsies obtained percutaneously to follow the treatment histopathologically. Type I dysplasia was seen in the smears from seven days after initiation, neoplastic nodules appeared later, and carcinoma cells were present after 15 weeks. Quantitative and cytochemical measurements of liver GGT activity showed an increase at the first sampling (two days after starting the treatment) and remained high thereafter. Serum analyses after 56 days of treatment also demonstrated a measurable increase in GGT activity.

In another study on the relationship of early histochemical changes in liver to carcinogenesis, Butler and colleagues (Butler and Hempsall, 1981; Butler et al., 1981) found that GGT and G6PD were elevated in basophilic hepatocyte foci after six weeks of treatment with 5 ppm AFB_1. The lesions were termed irreversible, based on the eventual development of malignancy when the animals were kept for one year after treatment. Histochemical changes that occurred in foci at three weeks, which reverted on termination of the treatment without neoplasia having developed, were starvation-resistant intracellular glycogen and depletion of G6P, succinate dehydrogenase, aniline hydrogenase, ATPase, and AP.

Harada et al. (1976) gave N-OH-FAA to rats in the diet continuously for 19 weeks; other rats received AFB_1 for seven weeks, the normal diet for 24 weeks, and AFB_1 for five more weeks. With N–OH–FAA, bile duct proliferation occurred after four weeks, hyperplasia after 16 weeks, and carcinomas after 36 and 56 weeks; with AFB_1, atypical focal changes were not seen for 36 weeks. GGT was histochemically affirmed in tumor cells and in proliferating bile ducts, including oval cells. Serum GGT was measurably elevated with N–OH–FAA after 16 weeks, but a longer period was required with AFB_1. The difference in response to N–OH–FAA and AFB_1 may have been due to the different regimens or doses used in the study.

A rise in liver GGT activity during treatment of rats with a chemical is not unequivocal evidence of hyperplasia that will lead to neoplasia. Fukushima et al. (1979) reported elevations in serum GGT in rats given 4,4'-diaminophenyl-urethane (a weak hepatocarcinogen) in the diet for 40 weeks, which they ascribed to proliferation of bile ductular cells, unrelated to neoplasia but histologically resembling what follows bile duct ligation or treatment with α-naphthyliso-cyanate. While GGT may be regarded as an indicator for cholestasis, some investigators consider it to be unreliable and relatively unresponsive in animal studies (Clampitt, 1978). Consequently, there are likely to be fewer false positives with GGT as an early marker for carcinogenesis in rats than might be expected from clinical surveys. When they occur the matter can be resolved by histopathologic examination.

These observations on GGT would lead one to the conclusion others (for example, Boelsterli, 1979) have reached--that GGT is a useful early marker of neoplasia in animal studies. To make use of this, one might consider assaying for its presence routinely during or after a 90-day "subchronic" study to support the need for long-term bioassay on a test chemical for carcinogenicity. For GGT to be useful and cost-effective in this way, however, suspected carcinogens must produce a change, detectable histochemically as GGT-positive foci or in serum within this time frame. For weak carcinogens, this may pose a problem. Higher doses of carcinogen or longer observation periods, such as four to eight weeks of recovery for some treated groups at the end of the subchronic study, might increase the sensitivity of this assay for early GGT changes. Alternatively, a promoter or cocarcinogen may be used with additional test groups to speed up carcinogenesis so that the effects of weaker carcinogens can be detected unequivocally within the customary 90-day study period.

The usefulness of GGT as a general preneoplastic marker would depend on the similarity of the carcinogenic process in other organs to that in the liver, something that has not been fully investigated. In this respect, it is interesting that 1,2-dimethylhydrazine-induced colon cancer in adult rats has been reported to yield highly elevated GGT activity when compared to homologous normal tissue (Fiala et al., 1977). Serum GGT levels may also enable the discrimination between normal and some neoplastic lymphoid cells (Novogrodsky et al., 1976; Culvenor et al., 1981) and aid in identifying chemically induced mammary adenocarcinomas (Sachdev et al., 1980).

In contrast to the rat, results with GGT in the mouse are somewhat inconclusive. Fiala and Fiala (1973) found that o-AAT given in the diet to mice for 70 to 80 days gradually increased liver GGT up to more than 10-fold, comparable to that obtained with feeding 3'-MeDAB or 2-AAF to rats for the same length of time; many hyperplastic nodules were present in the mouse liver. The GGT activity was doubled as early as four weeks after the treatment was started but was not present in spontaneously formed tumors in mice, a finding that was confirmed by a different laboratory (Jalanko and Ruoslahti, 1979) in a similar study with the same chemical. Kitagawa et al. (1980b) reported finding many GGT-positive foci or nodules in the livers of DEN-treated mice, although the tumors themselves at sacrifice were virtually all negative. Lipsky et al. (1981) found that foci, adenomas, and carcinomas in the liver of mice fed safrole in their diet all exhibited GGT-positive and G6P-negative properties, were resistant to Fe uptake histochemically, and ATPase levels were unchanged in these lesions relative to normal tissues. The GGT activity in the cells was variable; most occurred along the canalicular membranes, with some in the cytoplasm. In a more comprehensive survey with a variety of other enzyme markers, serum GGT was unchanged either by carcinogens or noncarcinogens whereas electrophoresis of plasma esterases discriminated between the two groups (Tyndall et al., 1978). In mice fed a diet containing griseofulvin for four to 17 months, nodules were low in GGT (Goldfarb et al., 1980), but increased plasma-membrane-bound ALP was demonstrated histochemically in all three types of foci. These lesions were interpreted to be preneoplastic; the more-developed Type 3 nodules were determined to be malignant.

In a third feeding study involving a chlorinated hydrocarbon pesticide, ALP and G6P were identified as good markers for mouse hepatic nodules, but GGT stained irregularly in these lesions (Essigmann and Newberne, 1981). These variations in GGT response may relate to differences in strain, test chemical, methodology, or other factors. They need to be resolved if GGT is to be considered as promising a marker for chemical-induced preneoplasia in mice as it is in rats.

Recent studies by Solt (1981) with DMBA suggest that GGT may serve as a preneoplastic marker for chemical carcinogenesis in the hamster buccal pouch, suggesting a more general scope for GGT in terms of species and type of experimental cancer. Support for the use of GGT activity as a specific and sensitive marker comes also from in vitro cell transformation studies on a variety of epithelial cell lines (Gerber et al., 1981; Shimada et al., 1980; Dolbeare et al., 1980; San et al., 1979) and on cells isolated from hyperplastic nodules and malignant lesions (Laishes et al., 1978). This marker is not induced in all transformed cell lines, however (Montesano et al., 1980; Sakakibara and Tsukada, 1980), indicating the phenotypic diversity of tumors.

Human Studies: Adequate information on which to assess GGT's potential as a preneoplastic marker in animal studies exists; its value in clinical medicine will be surveyed in less depth.

Despite early interest in GGT as a clinical marker, it has not gained widespread acceptance in the diagnosis of human cancer. A number of early reports suggested that it has value for the detection of liver metastasis (Braun et al., 1977; Balinsky, 1980; Schwartz, 1978), but Kim and his associates (1977) found GGT of questionable value for this application. While GGT produced the lowest false negatives of all the enzyme markers studied, it had a high rate of false positives (35%). Its utility improved when it was used with 5'-Nase, but the combination still correctly identified only 67% of patients with liver metastasis. ALP can be effective in predicting metastasis postoperatively when combined with other markers such as CEA and GGT and/or clinical examination and chest X-rays (Schwartz, 1976; Coombes et al., 1980; Coombes et al., 1981).

GGT has also been cited to be of value when used with ALP, LDH, and SGOT for predicting hepatic metastases in patients with gastrointestinal cancer (Huguier and Lacaine, 1981), with CEA for differentiating metastatic tumors in the uvea from primary uveal melanomas (Michelson et al., 1977), or with CEA and 5'-Nase to detect hepatic metastasis and for following therapy in bronchogenic carcinoma (Coombes et al., 1978).

Some investigators did not consider GGT to be useful in the early stages of disease or in discriminating benign from malignant tumors, and they did not recommend it for routine medical diagnosis (Cowen et al., 1978; Beck et al., 1978). A high incidence of false positives can be obtained because GGT also responds to cholestasis, mal-absorption, chronic alcoholism, hepatitis, myocardial infarction, neurological disease, and drug abuse (Ideo et al., 1972; Brunner and Schiller, 1977; Chaimoff et al., 1975; Goldberg and Martin, 1975; Braun et al., 1977; Evstigneeff et al., 1973; Schwartz, 1978). Also, it is sensitive to toxic liver damage caused by drug therapy, which could overshadow malignancy (Braun et al., 1977; Korsten et al., 1974; Warwas et al., 1977). This nonspe-cificity is not critical in rodent studies because of the lower hepatic content of GGT (Hagerstrand, 1973). Thus, canalicular GGT activity increases in man following biliary obstruction, whereas it is hardly affected in the rat (Hagerstrand, 1973). Correlating GGT with neoplasia in humans also may be complicated by the heterogeneity of other oncodevelopmental markers (Neuwald et al., 1980; Gerber and Thung, 1980).

GGT has been considered as a marker for tumors in tissues other than the liver. With colonic adenocarcinomas, GGT (and other oncodevelopmental enzymes) is appreciably ele-vated (Herzfeld and Greengard, 1980; Fiala et al., 1977); it is sometimes useful for early diagnosis of liver metas-tases, particularly together with CEA, and may help to investigate the evolution of colorectal cancer (Schwartz, 1978; Fiala et al., 1977). Its correlation with primary ovarian and cervical cancers is poor, even when combinations of markers are used (Dobryszycka et al., 1979; Malkin et al., 1978). GGT is present in human nephroblastomas (Wise and Muller, 1976), but it is much lower in other malignant renal tumors than in healthy tissue (Hagerstrand, 1973; Mattenheimer, 1977; Hautmann, 1979). In renal cancer, urinary GGT may be increased by nononcogenic disorders and drug treatments, as is the case with liver (Braun et al., 1977). These contrasting results suggest that it might be a useful indicator for renal cancer but only when complemented by other markers. One survey of 276 patients indicated little value for its use in early leukemias (Roberts et al., 1978).

Separation and analysis of GGT isozymes from liver and serum by polyacrylamide and agarose gel electrophoresis has been helpful in diagnosing hepatobiliary diseases, including malignancies of the liver and/or pancreas, in patients (Fujisawa et al., 1976; Kojima et al., 1980a; Suzuki, 1981; Hetland et al., 1975; Sawabu et al., 1980; Sawabu et al., 1978). Up to 13 different GGT bands were identified, but their usefulness in the early identification of disease is not yet established. [Isozyme analysis of GGT in rat breast can distinguish malignant from normal tissue (Jaken and Mason, 1978); similar analyses of liver and kidney have been proposed. This adds little in terms of detection in animal studies.]

Alkaline Phosphatase

The physiologic role of ALP is not adequately resolved (Tietz, 1976b). It is present in a variety of tissues but is highest in bone. It has been particularly valuable in identifying bone cancer (Schwartz, 1978).

Animal Studies: There has been far more interest in ALP as a marker for tumors in man than in animals. There are few animal studies in the recent literature on this subject. Feron and Kruysse (1977) studied the effects of exposing Syrian hamsters to acrolein vapor combined either with intratracheal instillation of BP or subcutaneous injection of DEN for 52 weeks. Animals were killed after 81 weeks. The "acrolein-only" group evidenced some toxic signs, including rhinitis with hyper- and metaplasia of the epithelium of the nasal cavity, after 52 weeks. After 81 weeks, respiratory tract tumors were present in the BP and DEN groups; acrolein did not enhance the effect. ALP was of no value in this study as an indicator of the presence of tumors.

Sugar et al. (1980) conducted a time-course study in which rats were given MNNG in the drinking water. Groups were killed every third week for up to 110 weeks and examined histologically. Regenerative hyperplasia in the stomach was seen almost at once, adenomatous hyperplasia (dysplasia) was seen after 23 weeks, and carcinomas were seen starting at about week 63. Eventually, 30 of 52 treated animals

developed carcinomas. Liver-type (nonplacental) ALP isozyme was detected in normal gastric cells, in atypical
hyperplasia, and in carcinomas, whereas the placental-type
(Regan) isozyme appeared only in the proliferating cells,
not in normal cells. Therefore, the latter isozyme was
considered indicative of malignant transformation. Miki
et al. (1980) reported that all MNNG-induced carcinomas had
ALP activity from "several" to 100 times higher than that
in surrounding tissue, and the induced ALP isozyme from the
metaplastic mucosa of rat stomach had properties similar
to its human counterpart. In a third study in which rats
received MNNG continuously for 104 weeks and then were sacrificed, ALP-positive foci were detected in gastric sites
containing very early tumors (not visible by other means)
and in areas of intestinal metaplasia (Morgan et al., 1981)
in a dose-dependent manner. Because time-dependent studies
were not conducted and no clear-cut carcinomas were found,
it could not be concluded that these foci represented preneoplastic lesions (Morgan et al., 1981).

These findings are not surprising in the light of other
reports of close correlations between ALP activity and
numbers of tumor cells. For example, mice with subcutaneous tumor implants exhibited a semilogarithmic relationship
between serum ALP activity and the number of osteosarcoma
cells; it was sensitive to more than 2×10^6 cells, an
otherwise undetectable population (Hiramoto et al., 1977).
In another study in which 1×10^6 osteosarcoma cells were
injected, serum ALP elevations occurred within five to ten
days and were closely correlated with tumor growth (Ghanta
et al., 1980). These reports suggest that serum ALP can
indicate the approximate size of disseminated and localized
tumors, but the indicator is not sensitive enough to pick
up very early localized tumors (Ghanta et al., 1976). In
rats, serum ALP was not significantly increased until the
transplanted tumor was palpable (Ingleton et al., 1979).
The differing ALP sensitivities may reflect species
differences.

Various other types of tumors have elevated ALP activity.
MNU-induced rat bladder tumors contained ALP localized as
a continuous layer around the cells, which contrasts with
its presence in the plasma membrane of basal and intermedi-
ate epithelial cells from normal adult rat bladder (Wilson
and Hodges, 1979). Discrete ALP-staining foci developed
in the former but not the latter after two weeks to two

months in culture. After culturing MNU-induced tumors, ALP levels were not higher than in those of normal bladder cells similarly cultured but they were higher in cultures of SV40-transformed WI-38 cells than in those of normal cells (Dolbeare et al., 1980). In the latter case, ALP and aryl amidase (lower activity) were the only two enzymes affected of the ten measured, including GGT. Cultured mouse B-lymphoma cell lines also exhibited an ALP elevation (Culvenor et al., 1981), but, overall, there appears to be considerable heterogeneity in ALP among various cell lines (Wilson and Hodges, 1979).

ALP has been proposed as a useful histochemical marker for nodular proliferative and neoplastic lesions in the mouse liver because it is present in Types 1, 2, and 3 foci after treatment over four to 17 months with a diet containing griseofulvin as an inducer (Goldfarb et al., 1980). The authors caution that their observations may apply only in the mouse. Others also consider ALP a good marker for mouse hepatic nodules, but, in these studies, ALP activity was decreased, possibly because of the toxic effects of the chlorinated hydrocarbon tested at the high dose (Essigmann and Newberne, 1981). Butler and Hempsall (1978) found ALP activity elevated in phenobarbitone-induced mouse liver nodules.

ALP does not appear to be similarly useful for the detection of liver hyperplasia in rats before carcinogenesis. Tatematsu et al. (1977), in a histochemical study of hyperplastic nodules formed in rat livers after treatment with several carcinogens, found that ALP was poorly defined in both nonhyperplastic and hyperplastic regions, whereas GGT and ATPase were considered to be good markers. Further, tissue ALP in rats exposed to vinyl chloride for three to four weeks was not significantly changed, whereas marker enzymes such as G6P and G6PD were affected (Du et al., 1979). This is unfortunate, because ALP changes due to other hepatic lesions, such as bile duct obstruction or hyperplasia from noncarcinogens, are not as likely to generate false positives in rodents as they are in humans (Ideo et al., 1972). However, even carcinogens may produce ALP elevations in bile duct canaliculi, associated with tissue regeneration. Neither are these changes specifically referable to oncogenesis in endothelial or other liver cells (Fukushima et al., 1979; Norpoth et al., 1980).

Human Studies: ALP is recognized as a clinical marker for
osteosarcoma (Schwartz, 1978; Fishman, 1974). When metastases appear from elsewhere, the greatest elevations in
serum are in patients with osteoblastic bone lesions. In
one survey, tissue levels of ALP in primary osteosarcomas
were positively correlated with the prognosis for pulmonary
metastases (Levine and Rosenberg, 1979).

The enzyme may have value for recognition of liver metastases also. Total ALP level in conjuction with other
indicators was considered potentially useful in monitoring
metastases postoperatively from breast cancer (Coombes et
al., 1977; Coombes et al., 1981), from colorectal cancer
(Tartter et al., 1981), from gastric cancer (Kojima et al.,
1979), from bronchogenic carcinomas (Coombes et al., 1978),
and from other malignancies (Ho et al., 1979). However, Kim
et al. (1977) demonstrated in their survey of four commonly
used serum indicators that ALP was not as good as 5'-Nase in
predicting hepatic metastases. Furthermore, certain investigators found that ALP was better than other serum indicators for the absence of hepatic metastasis than for its
presence in patients with gastrointestinal cancer (Huguier
and Lacaine, 1981). Likewise, lung adenocarcinomas can
produce serum ALP elevations without evidence of metastases
(Sells et al., 1979). Significantly higher ALP levels have
also been reported in patients with precancerous conditions
in the larynx than in normal controls (Lisiewicz et al.,
1978).

Generally, serum ALP has not been an effective marker for
primary tumors other than osteosarcomas. In breast cancer,
multivariate analyses (using several other common tumor
antigens, proteins, and enzymes, including ALP) were unable
to separate high-risk groups from those with benign breast
disease (Cowen et al., 1978). ALP and GGT levels were not
affected in the early stages of breast malignancies (Cowen
et al., 1978), but they may be useful in monitoring recurrence (Lee et al., 1980a). Serum ALP was not particularly
sensitive in detecting ovarian malignancies (Dobryszycka et
al., 1979; Burrows, 1980). ALP, along with several other
markers, was elevated in the cyst fluid of high-grade cystic
intracranial tumors but could not be used to distinguish
low-grade malignancies from benign tumors (Pullicino et al.,
1979). Thirteen patients with hepatocellular carcinomas
had tumor cells that stained intensely for GGT but were
deficient in ALP and other esterase activities (Uchida et
al., 1981).

In cases of fibrous dysplasia with malignant degeneration, elevated urine ALP often is found, usually associated with osteosarcomas (Campanacci et al., 1979). Urinary ALP has been helpful in conjunction with LDH in detecting renal carcinomas (Amador et al., 1963). Urinary ALP has not been useful for monitoring chemotherapy in acute leukemia (Posey et al., 1979).

Isozyme analysis of ALP is potentially more valuable for human cancer than is total serum ALP measurement (Schwartz, 1978; Fishman, 1974). A number of variants have been described (Fujisawa et al., 1976; Fishman, 1979). An attempt is made here only to identify instances in which isozyme analysis appears to improve the specificity and sensitivity of the ALP marker for the early detection of neoplasia.

Placental alkaline phosphatase (PLAP) isozyme has been extensively surveyed as a general cancer marker. Early reports on several hundred cancer patients were discouraging because of the low percentage of true positives (Stolbach et al., 1969; Nathanson and Fishman, 1971; Statland, 1981). Cadeau et al. (1974), in a larger survey, found it present in less than 10% of patients with various cancers (and in 2% of the serum of normal subjects), precluding its use as a general diagnostic screen. Other reviewers also noted that PLAP gives a low correlation with cancer and a large number of false positives (Tormey et al., 1979; Rochman, 1978).

However, Cadeau et al. (1974) were among the first to note a much higher occurrence of elevated PLAP activity in the serum of women with tumors of the reproductive tract, the breast, and the bladder than in cancer patients as a whole. In a more recent survey (Bhattacharya and Barlow, 1979; Fishman et al., 1975), the predictivity of the Regan isozyme (variant of PLAP) was much higher for ovarian adenocarcinomas (43%) and testicular carcinomas (42%) than reported above. The Nagao isozyme was almost twice as predictive for ovarian cancer when measured in ascitic fluid, but it yielded a large percentage of false positives (35%). In serum PLAP measurements of more than 1000 patients, about the same percentage of true positives was obtained for various gynecologic cancers (ovarian, cervical, and endometrial), with the percentage of false positives ranging from only 2% for ovarian carcinomas to 12% for carcinomas of the cervix (Haije et al., 1979). PLAP was considered

to be a better tumor marker than CEA for the former. These
findings are compared with those of Tottori (1979), who
observed that PLAP was a much poorer marker for most gynecologic malignancies than CEA and was comparable to AFP.
For ovarian carcinomas, CEA and PLAP were complementary
and reflected tumor burden, but with cervical carcinomas,
PLAP was found to be positive more often with minimal
disease (Malkin et al., 1978). This observation implies
difficulties of drawing inferences about early signs of
carcinoma from PLAP levels. Some of the findings with PLAP
may result from the presence of more than one phenotype of
placental ALP (Fishman et al., 1976). PLAP was suggested
as a useful marker for testicular tumors (seminomas), but
in advanced cases the best correlation was 60%, and the
percentage of false negatives for early or late tumors was
always high (45 to 65%), negating use of the isozyme for
screening (Wahren et al., 1979).

The value of serum PLAP for detection of some other tumor
types is less equivocal. It is insensitive for the diagnosis of bronchogenic carcinomas when relied on solely,
even though the Regan isozyme may be present in the tumor
(Coombes et al., 1978; Rochman, 1978; Rosen et al., 1975).
No clear relationship between ALP isozyme (Nagao type) and
intestinal metaplasia and gastric carcinomas has been found
(Fujisawa et al., 1976). It was not elevated in stage D
adenocarcinomas of the prostate (Broder et al., 1977), a
result similar to that reported above (Cadeau et al., 1974);
and AP had superior sensitivity (Beckley et al., 1980).
Chu et al. (1979) did report that the isozyme was present
in 18% of patients with stage D prostatic cancer, a frequency similar to the 22% average found by other investigators for most other tumor types. These investigators
noted that reproducing values in some patients from month
to month was difficult. The variability might be related
to gene expression at different phases of trophoblastic
development, as Fishman et al. (1976) found with ALP in
human cancer tissues. The predictivity of PLAP for any
of these tumors appears low and may be associated in part
with a poor correlation between serum and tumor levels of
ALP--e.g., ALP-1 in hepatomas (Toshitsugu et al., 1978).

Recent reports of novel ALP isozymes might hold more promise. For example, certain ALP isozyme activities were present in 90% or more of the patients with metastatic liver
cancer; the isozyme's origins are unclear because they were
not found in the hepatomas (Toshitsugu et al., 1978; Viot

et al., 1979). There was, however, a high number of false
positives (almost 20% attributable to cholestasis), but the
isozyme was not seen in normal subjects (Viot et al., 1979).
Bone isozyme was considered to be a more sensitive indicator
of metastatic adenocarcinomas of the prostate than was
total serum ALP activity (Chu et al., 1980). Koett et al.
(1979a,b) reported that a unique isozyme from patients with
liver malignancy associated with extrahepatic and/or intrahepatic cholestasis migrates faster than the "fast isozyme"
of Ehrmeyer et al. (1978). In electrophoresis on cellulose
acetate the isozyme appears most frequently in patients
with neoplastic diseases involving the liver. In a large
study (1692 patients), measurements of the fast-moving,
homoarginine-sensitive isozyme in serum recently revealed
that 58% of the patients with untreated or recurrent cancer
had the isozyme, in contrast to 11% with illnesses other
than cancer (Davis et al., 1981). These results were
equivalent to those in which CEA was used as the diagnostic
marker. Interestingly, a much greater elevation in serum,
fast-moving, ALP isozyme activity was found in patients with
breast, colorectal, and lymphomatous cancers than in those
with lung or gynecologic tumors (Davis et al., 1981). The
predictivity, however, remains low, and the isozyme is also
somewhat elevated in the sera of control patients with dia-
betes mellitus.

A slowly migrating, high-molecular-weight, altered form of
PLAP isozyme has been detected in JAR choriocarcinoma cells
in culture (Neuwald and Brooks, 1981). Cha et al. (1975)
also report a slowly moving band among PLAP isozymes in
sera; it exhibited an excellent correlation with the presence of pancreatic cancer (15 of 16 cases).

Neumann et al. (1976) reported that certain leukocytes also
contain a unique ALP that, unlike normal ALP isozymes, does
not hydrolyze S-substituted phosphate monoesters effectively
and may be a useful diagnostic tool in lymphoproliferative
diseases. Cytochemical studies indicated that a low percentage of the different non-Hodgkin lymphomas stained positively for ALP but that such cases did not constitute a
separate entity (Poppema et al., 1981). ALP isozymes from
these hematopoietic tumors are similar in most respects to
the placental Regan form (Damle et al., 1979). In a recent
survey of several different markers and various leukemias,
N-alkaline phosphatase was detected solely in lymphoid leukemic blast cells and was the most general of the markers

surveyed (Sakamoto et al., 1979). However, results reported
by others (Kelly et al., 1979) in diagnosing chronic lymphocytic leukemia are contradictory; questions about the existence of the marker need to be resolved. Other investigators
(Orlando et al., 1980) have claimed better success in the
diagnosis of chronic granulocytic leukemia using α-naphthyl-
acetate and α-naphthylbutyrate substrates. The group evaluated was small and needs to be expanded.

In summary, ALP is valuable principally for detecting osteosarcomas, its value as a test for liver metastasis is uncer-
tain, and it cannot be used currently as a general tumor
marker. Isozyme analysis is likely to improve detection of
some tumors, but inconsistent observations call for further
study. ALP isozyme analysis is complex and may contribute
to the varying results found by different laboratories. New
discoveries are enticing and encourage further work to sim-
plify and refine specificity and then sensitivity. The
complexity of such analyses as now performed suggests that
the routine use of ALP isozyme analysis in animal studies
would be costly.

MISCELLANEOUS ENZYMES

Several fairly common enzymatic indicators of hepatic disease have been reported to be useful for diagnosing cancer.
Although not usually classified as markers, their potential
value in the early detection of cancer is discussed in this
section. The enzymes include GOT (AST), GPT (AAT), GDH,
G6P, LAP, GDH, SDH, GDAP, glutaminase, and arginase.

Animal Studies

GOT and GPT: The transaminases GOT and GPT are clinical
indicators of lesions, particularly of the liver and the
heart when serum activity is elevated, and of the kidney
and urinary tract when urinary GOT levels are high. Because
liver necrosis is thought by some to be associated with
early steps in carcinogenesis, the correlation of liver
enzyme measurements in serum with preneoplastic lesions in
animals has been evaluated (Ying et al., 1980). Thus, various doses of nitrosamines combined with partial hepatectomy
were found to release GPT and SDH into rat serum concurrent
with the generation of neoplastic foci. When a choline-
deficient diet was used to exert an additional promoting
action with DEN as the initiator, serum GOT measurements

correlated well with the development of putative preneoplastic tissues (Sells et al., 1979). Because enzyme determinations in serum are more economical than cytochemical measurements, further work to assess the generality of this marker in available rat liver foci tests may be justified.

Serum transaminase levels are elevated in almost all chemical insults that cause liver cell necrosis, whether or not the chemicals are carcinogens. This would pose a major complication if these enzymes were to be used in conjunction with more tumor-specific markers to distinguish carcinogens in animal toxicity studies. For example, in a study in mice with a variety of carcinogens and noncarcinogens, serum GOT and serum LDH were elevated in all cases, whereas electrophoretic analyses of serum esterases exhibited altered profiles with the carcinogens only (Tyndall et al., 1978). Thus, GOT as an aid to identifying potential carcinogens in animals may be redundant if esterase analysis is sensitive enough. Also, noncarcinogens can produce histologic evidence of injury in the absence of measurable changes in enzyme activities (Nievel et al., 1976). Perhaps animal serum GPT and GOT are not more sensitive indicators of liver necrosis for many chemicals than is histopathologic examination (Grice, 1972; Cornish, 1971). This shortcoming must apply to carcinogenicity studies as well. For example, in a three- to four-week inhalation study with vinyl chloride, liver injury was detected by measuring G6P and G6PD activities in tissue homogenates and subcellular fractions after 70 to 140 hours of exposure, but serum transaminase levels were unchanged (Du et al., 1979). In this study, the enzyme changes correlated with changes in the endoplasmic reticulum confirmed under the electron microscope but were not observable at this stage by light microscopy.

G6P: G6P, a membrane-bound enzyme in the liver and kidney that hydrolyzes glucose-6-phosphate to glucose and phosphate (Hagerstrand, 1973), is released by hepatotoxins that cause necrosis (Platt and Cockrill, 1969), and by some carcinogens (Du et al., 1979), even within hours of treatment. These changes appear well before hyperplastic nodules can be detected, as they do when rats are given DEN in their drinking water (Curtin and Snell, 1980). However, G6P does not appear to be generally reliable for detection of hepatotoxins in rats. Crampton et al. (1977a,b) used changes in G6P activity in liver tissue to discriminate between transient induction of microsomal enzymes, liver damage, and nodular hyperplasia in rats exposed to phenobarbitone, BHT, safrole, or Ponceau MX in long-term studies in which tumors were not formed. Nievel et al. (1976) failed to find G6P useful in short-term studies with PB, BHT, and coumarin, despite histologic evidence of liver damage.

In contrast, mice given safrole in their diet for up to 75 weeks produced Fe-resistant foci after 24 weeks, hepatocellular adenomas with altered histochemical enzyme profiles (including G6P deficiency) after 36 weeks, and carcinomas that stained GGT-positive and G6P-negative after 52 to 75 weeks (Lipsky et al., 1981). A milder decrease in G6P was seen in areas of hepatocytomegaly surrounding the lesions.

G6P-deficient foci of hepatocytes have been found in eight-week-old mice given a single intraperitoneal injection of DEN shortly after birth; such foci were retained in the nodules and hepatomas that developed later (Moore et al., 1981). In mice, all DEN-induced foci were G6P-deficient. Ohmori et al. (1981) found that most spontaneous and BP-induced neoplasias in mice were G6P-deficient, in contrast to ATPase and GGT, which required PB promotion for optimal changes. Essigmann and Newberne (1981) also concluded that G6P activity was apparently a good marker for hyperplastic nodules in the mouse.

However, measurements of G6P activity in nodules and surrounding parenchyma in rats treated with 2-AAF showed only a halving of the activity, which, if it is directly extrapolatable to serum changes, is too insensitive to be useful (de Gerlache et al., 1980). The G6P activity of human hepatocellular carcinomas, like their counterparts in experimental carcinogenesis, is either absent or low (Uchida et al., 1981; Gerber and Thung, 1980; Gerber et al., 1981). There is also significant heterogeneity of enzyme phenotypes in human carcinomas (Gerber and Thung, 1980); adenomas, too, display abnormal enzyme patterns. In other carcinomas (e.g., of the uterine cervix) also, loss of G6P activity has been observed (Dutu et al., 1980). The cytoenzymatic techniques employed were not recommended for routine screening tests, and the fact that the G6P activity is lost rather than acquired by the modified cells suggests that its measurement in serum (Elder et al., 1972) would be too insensitive for use in clinical diagnosis.

Other Enzymes: Leucine aminopeptidase (LAP) is a marker for cholestasis that correlates well with changes in GGT in humans, but it is less sensitive than GGT and ALP in the rat (Ideo et al., 1972). The enzyme has apparently not been evaluated as a marker for cancer in animals. There are no indications from clinical surveys that it would prove useful.

Glutaminase (K) has been identified as a potentially useful marker from its appearance in tumors similar to that in fetal tissue (Knox, 1976), but this lead has not been exploited. Arginase, pyrroline-5-carboxylate reductase, and other enzymes, many of which were related to ornithine metabolism, were evaluated for their ability to detect submaxillary gland tumors in rats, but were not found to be effective (Herzfeld and Raper, 1976). Nor was liver arginase as sensitive as other marker enzymes in identifying distant cancer in the rat (Herzfeld et al., 1980).

Glutamate dehydrogenase (GDH) has been proposed to be more sensitive and organ-specific for liver necrosis in some animal species (including rodents) than indicators like serum GOT and GPT traditionally used for that purpose (Clampitt, 1978). The little information on its value as a cancer marker is not encouraging for its use in the rodent. Thus, Herzfeld et al. (1980) cautioned that soluble GDH would not be as sensitive in rats as in humans. Curtin and Snell (1980), in their study with rats exposed to DEN in drinking water for up to 15 weeks, found that the GDH in rat liver nodules considered to be preneoplastic showed less histochemical change than other, more sensitive enzymes.

There is a report of highly increased GDH (and aminopeptidase) activities in a variety of human lung tumors (60 altogether) that may have clinical value (Ionescu et al., 1979), but their use as early markers remains to be demonstrated.

Sorbitol dehydrogenase (SDH) is conveniently measured in serum and has also been considered by some researchers to be a more sensitive indicator of liver cell necrosis in rodent studies than serum GPT and GOT (Cornish, 1971; Grice, 1972). For this reason, SDH level has been monitored in studies that attempt to relate acute hepatic necrosis to the induction of early stages of liver carcinogenesis by known carcinogens (Ying et al., 1981; Ying et al., 1980). Its value in detecting preneoplastic conditions is low for the same reason given for the serum transaminases: it cannot discriminate between injurious chemicals that induce neoplasia and those that do not. However, if serum GOT is a useful adjunct to mechanistic investigations using the rat liver foci model, GDH and SDH should be also.

GPAD reportedly compares favorably with GGT as an early indicator of hepatic cancer in animal studies (Kojima et al., 1980b,c), but its practical value is limited by its relative insensitivity. In rats fed 3'-MeDAB in the diet, serum GPAD and GGT activities increased before tumors appeared. Although the relative increase in GPAD activity was not as great as that of GGT, it occurred much earlier. The cellular distribution of GPAD shifted from the microsomal fraction to the supernatant fraction of hepatic cancer tissue, unlike GGT, which increased in both fractions. When gross tumors were present in the animals, GPAD in serum was double that in controls and lower in tumor tissues; the respective GGT increases were 20- and 50-fold (Kojima et al., 1980c).

The rat data with GPAD paralleled data obtained in the sera of cancer patients, in which the mean value for those with cancer was almost three times the normal mean value (Kojima et al., 1980a,b). Aminopeptidases and arylamidases in human liver, lung, and stomach cancers have immunologic and chromatographic differences that may, if present in sera (or tissue biopsies), be diagnostically useful, because the patterns may be organ-specific (Niinobe et al., 1979). In transformed WI-38 cells, GPAD activity was unchanged from that of the normal cell line, again a reflection of the relative insensitivity of qualitative criteria of this enzyme's activity as a marker (Dolbeare et al., 1980). Arylamidase levels, on the other hand, were greatly diminished in the transformed cells.

Other enzymes that show some potential as early tissue markers for preneoplastic lesions are serine dehydratase (Kitagawa, 1976) and pyrroline-5-carboxylate reductase (Herzfeld et al., 1980). Kitagawa (1976) found that hyperplastic areas in the livers of rats fed 2-AAF in the diet had marked deficiencies in β-glucuronidase and serine dehydratase during the development phase (weeks 6-9); a small group of larger lesions kept this deficiency throughout the observation period (18 weeks) and appeared to be more important for the eventual development of carcinomas. Unlike the situation in humans, the response of total pyrrolidine-5-carboxylate reductase in rat liver to distant cancers and loss of enzyme activity are less dependable indications of neoplasia because they may arise from nonspecific inactivation of catalytic functions (Herzfeld et al., 1980).

Tyndall et al. (1978) reported that plasma esterase activity profiles in mice changed within seven days of exposure to high concentrations of several carcinogens (including two that were not hepatocarcinogens) but were unchanged after exposure to high concentrations of weakly carcinogenic or noncarcinogenic compounds. The indicator change was more discriminatory than were measurements of the serum GOT or LDH.

Human Studies

Almost without exception, serum transaminases alone have not been useful in cancer diagnosis, but some clinicians have found them of value in conjunction with other markers. Thus, tissue GPT was not useful in identifying cancer patients with liver metastasis (Herzfeld et al., 1980), but combinations of GOT and other serum enzymes (GGT, ALP, and LDH) were said to increase the predictive value for the absence or presence of hepatic metastasis in patients with gastrointestinal cancer to 80 to 90% (Huguier and Lacaine, 1981). For the diagnosis of ovarian carcinoma, serum GOT-- alone or together with LDH or ALP--was not sensitive enough to be useful (Burrows, 1980), but when either serum GOT or GPT was used to supplement RNase, detection of nonmalignant and malignant ovarian tumors was greater than with any other single indicator or combination (Dobryszycka et al., 1979). For other types of cancers--e.g., breast, brain or CNS-- transaminase measurements have not been informative (Seiden- feld and Marton, 1978; Y. T. Lee et al., 1980; Hildebrand, 1973; Wasserstrom et al., 1981; Seidenfeld and Marton, 1979).

The value of LAP as a general screen for CNS, ovarian, and hepatic tumors and for intestinal metaplasia did not appear to be useful (Seidenfeld and Marton, 1979; Dobryszycka et al., 1979; Ideo et al., 1972; Warwas et al., 1977; Wasser- strom et al., 1981; Matsukura et al., 1979). A related peptidase, GPN, measured in the sera of patients with hepa- tobiliary disease (Hutchinson et al., 1981), was reported to be useful for detecting metastases and other hepatic lesions. Urinary arylsulfatase appears to be very effective for monitoring the response to antileukemic agents (Posey et al., 1979); its value for detecting early stages relative to that of other potential indicators would be of interest.

Soluble GDH was one of five enzymes found to be affected
in liver biopsies from cancer patients (Herzfeld et al.,
1980). Its activity dropped the most, to 20% of control
levels. Few other data exist by which to assess the diagnostic value of GDH for cancer or preneoplasia. Kim et
al. (1977) measured serum levels of GDH in their survey of
enzyme markers for liver metastases and estimated that its
predictivity would be low. Cytoenzymatic tests on malignant
cells in vaginal fluids did not show GDH to be useful in a
general screen (Dutu et al., 1980).

Investigators report that detecting neoplasia can be
improved by using a set of enzyme markers. Thus, Herzfeld
et al. (1980) found that the pattern of pyrroline-5-
carboxylate reductase and four other liver enzymes measurable in cancer hosts was not seen in any cancer-free patient
whether or not the latter had morphologic liver damage. The
group sizes were small, but the good correlation encourages
broadening the investigation. In another study, a set of
eight enzymes including pyrroline-5-carboxylate reductase
distinguished (1) neoplastic from nonneoplastic sections of
adult colon and (2) moderately or well-differentiated from
poorly differentiated pulmonary adenocarcinomas (Herzfeld
and Greengard, 1980). Several investigators have stressed
the value of larger sets of enzyme analyses because they
were more discriminating and sensitive indications of neoplasms than multivariate analysis of a few selected enzymes
(Knox, 1976).

Overall, the current clinical literature neither supports
nor refutes the observations made about the enzymes discussed in the preceding sections on animal studies. The
survey of Herzfeld et al. (1980) on 13 hepatic enzymes
involving various metabolic pathways showed several significant differences in their responsiveness to chemically
induced cancer in rats and its "spontaneous" occurrence in
humans (e.g., GDH, pyrroline-5-carboxylate reductase, ornithine aminotransferase). Other enzyme responses, in contrast, were similar in the two species. Such observations
limit the prospects of easy extrapolation from animal to
man and vice-versa.

RAT LIVER FOCI AS SCREENS

A variety of experimental models have evolved for the study
of the morphologic events leading to hepatocarcinogenesis

(Farber, 1980; Pitot and Sirica, 1980; Farber and Cameron, 1980; Weisburger and Williams, 1981; Pereira, 1982) (see Table V-1). They involve initiator and promoter combinations that increase the rate of formation of hyperplastic lesions and tumors (and/or their numbers). Interest in these models is augmented by the possibility that they may provide a relatively inexpensive and rapid means of identifying and classifying carcinogens (Anonymous, 1982; Bull and Pereira, 1982; Pereira, 1982).

In the earliest model for hepatocarcinogenesis, that of Peraino and his colleagues (see Farber and Cameron, 1980, p. 145), in which PB (or DDT) was used as a promoting agent and 2-AAF as the initiator, putative preneoplastic nodules, identified microscopically, occurred within 18 days in the livers of rats, and tumors appeared several months later. Several known carcinogens gave positive results with this model. Recently, it has been modified to use DEN as the initiating agent (given one day after birth) with PB administration begun at weaning. GGT was adopted as a putative marker for the development of foci (Peraino et al., 1981).

The model of Scherer, Emmelot, and co-workers (Scherer et al., 1972; Scherer and Emmelot, 1975, 1976) employed partial hepatectomy (PH) in female rats to increase the rate of cell proliferation. ATPase or G6P deficiency (or both) or glycogen persistence were used as histochemical markers to quantify early preneoplastic lesions.

A variant of this model developed by Pitot and co-workers combines PH and PB, and uses a combination of ATPase, G6P, and GGT as markers (Pitot, 1977; Pitot et al., 1978). With this model, a single intragastric dose of DEN produced enzyme-altered foci and hepatomas in rats after eight to ten months. Hyperplastic foci would probably have been evident sooner had time-course studies been performed. With this model, a number of potent promoters have been identified, including HBB (Jensen et al., 1982) and TCDD, with the induction period for tumors reduced to seven weeks (Pitot et al., 1980).

Solt and Farber (1976) and colleagues used a single or a few repeated doses of an initiating carcinogen, with PH and an additional carcinogen (such as 2-AAF or ethionine) at a level that produces cytotoxicity without tumor formation (Farber and Cameron, 1980). This tactic was based on the premise that sensitivity could be increased by inhibiting the proliferation of normal hepatocytes by using low doses

Table V-1

RAT LIVER FOCI SCREENS

Model	Initiator	Promoter	Weeks to Hyperplastic Lesions	References
1	2-AAF	PB	Several	Peraino et al., 1971 1975, 1977
	DEN	DDT		Ohde et al., 1979
	3'-MeDAB	BHT		
		γHCH		
		Prenatal or newborn	7	Peraino et al., 1981
2	DEN	PH	4	Scherer and Emmelot, 1975
	DMN			
	3'-MeDAB			
	AFB			
	Ethionine			

(Continued)

Table V-1 (Concluded)

Model	Initiator	Promoter	Weeks to Hyperplastic Lesions	References
3	DEN	PH + PB	~6	Pitot, 1977 Pitot et al., 1978
4	Various	2-AAF + PH + CCl$_4$	5	Solt and Farber, 1976 Solt et al., 1977 Tsuda et al., 1980
5	Various	CD-diet + PH ± PB	3-9	Takahashi et al., 1979

of a known carcinogen that would not lead to tumor
formation. The cocarcinogen-resistant cells would then
continue to grow under these conditions. Their model has
been modified to include a single treatment with CCl_4 during
the 2-AAF exposure phase (Tsuda et al., 1980: Tsuda and
Farber, 1980). The assay can take as few as six weeks for
definitive appearance of foci; GGT is used as the marker
of choice.

Diet manipulation has been used to shorten the latent period required for the appearance of hepatocellular carcinoma
after exposing rodents to known or suspected carcinogens
(Rogers and Newberne, 1975; Rogers, 1975; Mabuchi, 1979;
Thompson and Vladislava, 1981). The most promising scheme
is a choline-devoid diet which serves as a promoting
agent for suspected carcinogens. Using this procedure DL-
ethionine, azaserine, and 2-AAF produced hepatocellular
carcinomas in 50% or more of the tested rats within three
to six months (Shinozuka et al., 1978a,b; Lombardi and
Shinozuka, 1979). Enzyme-altered focus induction (GGT)
is also augmented by this manipulation, analogous to PB
promotion, with the foci appearing three to four weeks
after a single injection of either azaserine or DEN while
on a choline-devoid diet (Takahashi et al., 1979; Sells et
al., 1979). Plasma GGT correlated with the number of GGT-
positive foci but plasma AFP did not (Sells et al., 1979).

Tests or screens for promoters employ the same biochemical
markers as those for initiators, because the same endpoints
(foci, nodules and tumors) are sought. For example, with
DEN or 2-AAF as the initiator, together with PH, a short-
term screen (six to 16 weeks) for promoters has been proposed that uses GGT as the putative marker (Tatematsu et
al., 1977, 1979). Other markers that have been used to complement GGT, and sometimes instead of GGT, in these short-
term tests for preneoplastic foci are listed in Table V-2.

Several studies have shown that the hyperplastic foci are
heterogeneous with respect to any set of histochemical markers. With a single carcinogen (DEN or 2-AAF) and with GGT,
ATPase, and G6P used as markers, all possible phenotypes
have been found among hyperplastic foci (Pitot, 1977; Pugh
and Goldfarb, 1978; Pitot et al., 1978). Almost all G6P-
and ATPase-deficient foci were GGT-positive (Ogawa et al.,
1980), and GGT was the most common focus-associated marker
of the three (Farber and Cameron, 1980). Greater diversity is observed as foci progress to tumors (Ogawa et al.,

Table V-2

SOME HISTOCHEMICAL MARKERS OF HYPERPLASTIC FOCI

Histochemical Marker	Change	References
GGT	Increase	Pitot, 1977
Basophilia	Increase	Fiala and Fiala, 1973
DT-diaphorase	Increase	Schor et al., 1978
DNA synthesis	Increase	Ohde et al., 1979
Ornithine decarboxylase	Increase	Olson and Russell, 1980
PN-antigen (EH?)	Appearance	Okita and Farber, 1975
G6P	Decrease	Scherer and Emmelot, 1976
ATPase (canalicular)	Decrease	Scherer and Emmelot, 1978
Fe uptake	Decrease	Williams and Watanabe, 1978
Serine dehydratase	Decrease	Kitagawa and Pitot, 1975
β-Glucuronidase	Decrease	Kitagawa and Pitot, 1975
Glycogen (fasting)	Unchanged	Scherer and Emmelot, 1975

1980), but in studies carried out long enough for hepatocellular carcinomas to develop, the GGT-positive phenotype was
invariably present, even though one or two animals exhibited
some GGT-negative tumors (Pugh and Goldfarb, 1978). Thus,
the change in enzyme pattern in hyperplastic foci has been
suggested as an early reflection of carcinogenesis, although
experimental demonstration of the relationship is not conclusive (Pitot and Sirica, 1980).

The most active lesions, based on [^{3}H]-thymidine incorporation into DNA, were those in which changes in the levels
of all three enzyme markers (G6P, ATPase, and GGT) occurred
(Pugh and Goldfarb, 1978), but this correlation did not
extend to the carcinomas themselves (Goldfarb and Pugh,
1981). G6P is the least sensitive of the commonly used
markers for hyperplastic foci, probably because it is
changed in fewer phenotypes than are the other markers
(Hirota and Williams, 1979; Pitot et al., 1980; Pugh and
Goldfarb, 1978; Pitot et al., 1978; Goldfarb and Pugh,
1981; Ogawa et al., 1980). Because G6P-negative phenotypes
occur much less often than GGT-positive or ATP-negative
ones (Pugh and Goldfarb, 1978), some investigators consider
the latter to be better markers in the rat liver foci model
for carcinogenesis (Tatematsu et al., 1977). However, G6P
deficiency is an important characteristic of preneoplastic
lesions that progress to cancer (Pugh and Goldfarb, 1978;
Goldfarb and Pugh, 1982), but its analysis may be redundant
in the rat liver foci model. Similar considerations apply
to most of the other markers listed in Table V-2.

If research continues to seek a "most likely" pattern of
neoplastic development (Goldfarb and Pugh, 1982), GGT will
probably remain an indispensable marker of preneoplasia
in the rat. This will be true even if oval cells rather
than or in addition to hyperplastic foci should prove to
be precursors of nodule formation or tumors directly, as
Sell and Leffert (1982) propose, because GGT is found in
oval cells as well as in foci.

A mouse liver foci model does not yet exist. Cater et al.
(1982) applied the Peraino model to the mouse with DMN
instead of DEN as the initiator. The combination of a
single injection of DMN and a PB-containing diet commencing
at weaning resulted in the sequential development of GGT-
positive liver foci and nodules over a 16-week period that
were also Fe-resistant and morphologically similar to pre-
sumptive preneoplastic lesions in chemically induced rat

liver foci. Overt tumors were not found in any animals,
and treated animals were not held long enough to confirm
that tumors could be formed by the treatment. GGT can be
induced in hepatomas in mice by PB promotion, but it is
not regularly present in spontaneous tumors (Ohmori et al.,
1981; Williams et al., 1980).

The activities of GGT, ATPase, and G6P markers in human nodular "regenerative" hyperplasia and hepatocellular carcinomas have also been evaluated histochemically and found to
exhibit phenotypic diversity similar to that reported in the
rat (Gerber and Thung, 1980; Thung and Gerber, 1981; Uchida
et al., 1981). Some authors suggest that the similarity
indicates that the enzyme alterations during experimental
hepatocarcinogenesis are relevant to the human disease
(Gerber and Thung, 1980).

XENOBIOTIC METABOLIZING ENZYMES

Xenobiotic chemicals are metabolized by a group of relatively nonspecific enzymes (primarily found in the liver but
also in other tissues), usually in two phases. In Phase I,
polar-reactive groups added to the molecule increase its
water solubility; in Phase II, the Phase I product is conjugated with endogenous substrates to produce highly water-
soluble, excretable metabolites. Of the Phase I reactions,
the monooxygenase (MFO) transformations in the smooth endoplasmic reticulum are the best known. Cytochrome P450 is
the terminal oxidase of an enzyme complex that uses O_2 and
reducing equivalents to incorporate one of the oxygen atoms
into the xenobiotic substrate. NADPH-cytochrome c reductase
is a component of the microsomal electron transport chain
that supplies electrons to cytochrome P450.

The products of the Phase I metabolism pathways are often
unstable, reactive intermediates (such as epoxides or arene
oxides). These highly reactive epoxides [usually from the
metabolism by aryl hydrocarbon hydroxylase (AHH), a cytochrome P450-dependent MFO (Kouri et al., 1980)], may change
spontaneously to phenols, be converted enzymatically by
epoxide hydrolase (EH) (another Phase I enzyme, not P450-
dependent) to a dihydrodiol, or be conjugated with glutathione by soluble glutathione-S-epoxide transferase (a
Phase II enzyme). The dihydrodiols or phenols may also
be substrates for conjugation with glucuronide, sulfate,
or amino acids, or become monooxygenated a second time to
form a highly reactive diol-epoxide. The primary epoxides,

as well as the secondarily formed diol-epoxides, can bind covalently to critical cellular macromolecules, thereby leading to toxic effects, mutation, and cancer (Gielen et al., 1979).

The tissue concentrations of many of these enzymes are increased on initial exposure to xenobiotics; the concentrations of others may be reduced as a result of chemical-caused necrosis, for example. Thus, the enzymes critical to toxication or detoxication of xenobiotics are worth consideration as indirect indicators for carcinogens, even though they are not ordinarily detectable in sera or urine. The high metabolic capability of the liver, its large size, and the ease of obtaining liver samples make it the preferred organ for monitoring these enzyme systems.

The most promising biochemical marker among the Phase I and Phase II enzymes for use in the early detection of hepatocarcinogenesis is EH. As a key enzyme in the detoxification of the epoxides thought to be responsible for macromolecular damage that may lead to cancer, EH has been extensively studied in the livers of animals exposed to carcinogens. In all such studies, it was found to increase long before tumors formed [e.g., within one to five weeks (Griffin, 1981)]. For example, EH was increased in rat hyperplastic nodules produced by 2-AAF and persisted both in the nodules and hepatocellular carcinomas that developed after omission of the carcinogen, but not in nontumor tissue (Novikoff et al., 1979; Cameron et al., 1979). When measured in liver microsomes, it was also increased within four days after administration of five different classes of hepatocarcinogens--2-AAF, azo dye, DEN, AFB_1, or safrole (Cameron et al., 1979; Sharma et al., 1981). [Changes in microsomal EH activity after the administration of 2-AAF for three days to two weeks were related to known species and sex differences (rats and mice) in the carcinogenicity of this chemical (Graichen and Dent, 1982)]. EH was also six to ten times higher in rat livers following five-day oral administration of the hepatocarcinogens AFB_1, 2-AAF, DNT, 2,4-DAT, and DEN, whereas NADPH-cytochrome c reductase and other MFO activities were unchanged (Dent, 1980). The nonhepatocarcinogens tested, 3-MC and MNU, had no effect on EH, and the hepatotoxin bromobenzene produced only a mild increase. Hepatocarcinogens not capable of epoxidation (TA or ethionine) can also increase EH (Griffin, 1981). Nonhepatocarcinogens can be made to stimulate EH activity

with the aid of a promoter. Thus, dimethylhydrazine, a
colon carcinogen, increased liver EH activity when given
to rats within 12 hours after PH; administration of the
carcinogen without this manipulation produced no change
in EH (Cameron et al., 1979).

EH elevation is not unequivocal evidence for the eventual
appearance of malignancy. In early focal proliferative
lesions, over 90% of which were GGT-positive, EH staining
was variable when DEN was the initiator and 2-AAF and PH
the promotors. The majority of foci showed less staining
than surrounding hepatocytes (Enomoto et al., 1981). Two
weeks later, when the lesions were macroscopically visible,
almost all were EH-positive. Surrounding hepatocytes had
reduced EH staining. In nodules that had stopped proliferating and returned to their normal phenotype, GGT decreased,
but EH did not.

In another study, rats were given 10 to 20 mg/kg NNM daily
in drinking water (Kuhlmann et al., 1981). After 64 days,
the earliest time investigated, EH was prominent in distinct
liver cell islets but a reduction in ATPase was less apparent. After 94 days, increased EH and decreased ATPase were
clearly detectable and GGT began to appear. All three markers persisted, even after NNM had been discontinued for
up to 26 weeks. An interesting finding was the presence
of EH in benign tumors, although it was absent in malignant
tumors. Further, some (but not all) purely cholestatic
agents increased EH levels following short-term (two to
six weeks) administration (Thompson et al., 1982).

In the human studies reviewed, EH was detected in all samples of lungs having a diagnosis of cancer, and one sample
with tuberculosis also revealed levels in the range seen
for cancer patients (Greene and Jernstrom, 1980). No other
control patients were studied. In another study, EH was
measured in the lungs of smokers and of nonsmokers with
and without lung cancer (Lorenz et al., 1979). No significant difference was found in EH activity between noncancer
patients and nonsmokers, and patients with lung cancer;
the values for the two former groups fell within the range
noted for lung cancer patients in the study conducted by
Greene and Jernstrom (1980).

Using MFO inhibition as an indicator is limited largely
to changes in the liver, because it contains the most MFO-

mediated activity. Inhibition of activity, when associated
with hyperplasia in the liver, may be an early indication of
hepatotoxicity, as noted with safrole and the azo compound
Ponceaux MX (Crampton et al., 1977b). This hepatotoxicity
may be responsible for changes in the enzyme levels of
preneoplastic tissues. Thus, NADPH-cytochrome c reductase
and cytochrome P450 activities were decreased in hyperplastic nodules of the liver after treatment for 14 weeks with
2-AAF (Cameron et al., 1976), with ethionine (Gravela et
al., 1975), and with 3'-MeDAB (Oyanagui et al., 1974).
Greengard (1979) found that the reductase was also decreased
in the liver of rats with subcutaneous tumor implants, but
the change was less sensitive than that of other measured
enzymes (e.g., ornithine aminotransferase, glucokinase, or
GPT) and occurred only after the tumors became palpable.
Although more work is needed to identify the most sensitive
and specific set of markers and to expand these findings to
other types of tumors, reduced marker activity in the liver
rather than in serum may be a useful early indication of
extrahepatic neoplasia as well as of hepatocarcinogenesis;
thus, only one tissue need be monitored histochemically in
routine animal studies.

MFO activity may be induced by a wide variety of compounds
differing in structure and biologic activity (Crampton et
al., 1977a) and is usually accompanied by liver enlargement.
BHT and PB cause hypertrophy and hyperplasia of the liver
but no damage associated with release of lysosomal enzymes,
even after long-term treatment (Crampton et al., 1977a).
However, similar treatment with safrole, DDT, and dieldrin
induces not only MFO but also hepatic nodules. Thus, there
appears to be no predictable relationship between MFO induction and nodular hyperplasia (Crampton et al., 1977b).

Also, the early induction of AHH is not likely to serve as
a reliable indicator of hepatocarcinogenesis, except perhaps
when AHH is induced specifically by polyaromatic hydrocarbons. AHH, along with other MFOs, is decreased in hyperplastic nodules induced by 2-AAF in the liver (Cameron et
al., 1976). However AHH activity is increased before apparent tissue involvement. This response is most specific
for polyaromatic hydrocarbons such as BP in cigarette smoke
(Gielen et al., 1979; Uotila, 1977) and diesel exhaust (Lee
et al., 1980b), although it also occurs with other carcinogens such as AFB_1 (Singh and Clausen, 1980).

This inductive response also has been demonstrated in other
cell types in vitro or in vivo. AHH was increased in both
normal and neoplastic human breast epithelium in culture
in response to DMBA, BP, and BA (Greiner et al., 1980).
Lymphocytes and macrophages from patients with lung cancer
had higher AHH activity than did cells from noncancer
patients (Snodgrass et al., 1981). This inductive response
is transient, because AHH activity falls like that of other
MFOs when hyperplastic nodules form. Its importance as
an indicator is restricted to polyaromatic hydrocarbons.

SUMMARY ASSESSMENT

The principal criteria for assessing the foregoing indicators as early evidences of hepatic and renal carcinogenesis in animals are their specificity and sensitivity. If
serum and urine are to be monitored in short-term repeated
exposure studies, for example, preliminary evidence can
usually be verified by histopathologic examination of the
tissues upon sacrifice of the animals. If no histopathologic (or other) basis is found, but the marker is known
to be closely associated with preneoplastic events, further
testing of the inducing chemical may be warranted. When
liver and kidney tissues are examined histochemically, sensitivity for the detection of preneoplastic lesions (which
may not be discernible by the usual staining techniques)
becomes important. Unlike in human medicine, only a few
markers can be measured conveniently, reliably, and repro-
ducibly and be economically justifiable for screening chemicals and include also examination of tissues routinely, as
indicated. Relative to target organs, available indicators
are given primary importance in testing chemicals for oncogenicity in the context of specificity and sensitivity.

Available information indicates that there is no perfect,
generally predictive, tumor-specific marker among those
reviewed in this section for early detection of induced
carcinogenesis in animals. There are, however, sufficient
data to justify the continued use of γ-glutamyl transpeptidase (GGT), considered by many investigators to be the
most valuable marker for that purpose. GGT is found cyto-
chemically to be elevated in irreversible, hyperplastic foci
and nodules, lesions thought to be precursors of hepatomas
and hepatic carcinomas (Pereira, 1982). Although there is
considerable phenotypic diversity with some GGT-negative
tumors, we are not aware of a study in which a chemical

carcinogen that produced elevations of GGT in a substantial percentage of hepatocellular foci (usually about 90%) failed to produce carcinomas.

Hence, the probability that GGT analysis will generate false negatives in experimental carcinogenesis in the rat appears to be extremely low. However, false negatives may result if reliance is based solely on GGT elevation, as evidenced by the recent report of Rao et al. (1982), in which hyperplastic foci and nodules were GGT-negative in animals in which liver hepatocellular carcinomas (also GGT-negative) eventually appeared following prolonged treatment of Fischer 344 rats with a hypolipidemic chemical incorporated in their diet. Some false positives also may occur (Pereira, 1982), but the probability may be kept low by prudent selection of complementary markers and conscientious histologic examination of the livers at sacrifice.

The GGT marker is being applied routinely in rat liver foci tests in some laboratories using repeated or single-dose studies with test chemicals (without promoter or cocarcinogen). The latter types of studies may justify the cost of carrying out the adjunctive histochemical examination, because the liver is one of the most common target organs for carcinogens. Alternatively, the more economical serum analysis for GGT could be done with a likely reduction in sensitivity. If serum GGT is found to be elevated, the presence of preneoplastic liver lesions would be suspected.

There are some qualifications to the general applicability of GGT as a preneoplastic indicator that need to be resolved (Table V-3). The need for more definitive evidence for a precursor relationship between induced GGT-positive hyperplastic foci and carcinoma is a fundamental area in which progress is being made (Goldfarb and Pugh, 1982). Further, an understanding of the nature of the biphasic quantitative changes in liver GGT and their relationship to hepatocarcinogenesis needs to be clarified. Will changes that may be undetected appear with promoters? Also, can the contrasting results between mice and rats using GGT as a preneoplastic marker be explained? Finally, GGT may be a useful marker for tumors in organs other than the liver (e.g., colon, breast, and some lymphoid cell types). Can preneoplastic lesions be detected in these organs? According to the more extensive human clinical investigations, it appears that GGT may not turn out to be generally useful for this purpose, except as one of a battery of marker tests.

Dr Dahl

Centrax® (prazepam) (IV C)

5 mg, 10 mg and 20 mg capsules
10 mg scored tablet

PARKE-DAVIS
Div of Warner-Lambert Co
Morris Plains, NJ 07950

PD-R-2873-3-P (1-86)

Table V-3

POTENTIAL VALUE AS PRENEOPLASTIC OR EARLY NEOPLASTIC MARKER

Indicator	Potential	Qualifications
GGT	Excellent	1) May be limited to liver and a few other organs, i.e., specificity.
		2) Species limited.
ALP	Possible	1) Preneoplastic or early indicator in mouse only.
		2) Isozyme analysis sharpens interpretation.
		3) A general marker.
		4) How specific is it in animals for neoplasia.
EH	Possible	1) Association with malignancy equivocal.

ALP also has some promise as an early neoplastic marker for chemically induced carcinogenesis. Several studies, particularly with the mouse, indicate that it could be a useful histochemical marker of hepatic nodules and proliferative lesions that are thought to be precancerous. Changes in serum ALP (or its isozymes) might indicate the presence of small tumors and thus have broader utility than histochemical studies suggest. ALP may not be sufficiently specific for neoplasia, however; more information on its specificity and sensitivity in experimental carcinogenesis in various species is required to assess its potential. Also, the economy of urine enzyme analyses of ALP for kidney and bladder tumors in the rodent needs to be demonstrated.

EH is another cytochemical marker for hepatocarcinogenesis and has received more attention in experimental studies than ALP. It may be a suitable adjunct in screening for carcinogens in rat liver foci tests. Its activity is altered early during a carcinogenic process by a variety of test chemicals, including those not expected to be changed into epoxides. While some studies have shown that elevated EH persists in nodules and carcinomas, others failed to demonstrate an unequivocal relationship with malignancy. Consequently, this indicator may yield false positives unless methods can be developed to resolve the discrepancies.

In addition to the enzymes listed in Table V-3, GOT, GPT, GDH, SDH, LAP, GPAD, aminopeptidase, arginase, G6P, pyrroline-5-carboxylate reductase, arylamidase, methylene tetrahydrofolate reductase, transglutaminase, cytochrome P450, NADPH-cytochrome c reductase, aryl hydrocarbon hydroxylase, and other xenobiotic metabolizing enzymes were considered for their possible applications as early detectors of neoplasia. Interest is not strong in any of them at this time because none is either sufficiently specific or adequately sensitive relative to other markers such as GGT. They could be used however, as part of a large battery of tests to improve predictivity. Additional studies with some of these indicators, GDAP for example, may demonstrate high specificity and good sensitivity as preneoplastic markers with a larger number of chemicals and thus require an upgraded assessment of their efficacies.

VI

Glycosyltransferases

A.E. Brandt

INTRODUCTION

One of the most consistent observations associated with
tumorigenesis is the altered expression of cell-surface
glycolipid and glycoprotein carbohydrate structures. The
enzymes that catalyze the formation of oligosaccharide
structure, namely the glycosyltransferases, have been
studied in normal and tumor tissue and in the serum of
normal and tumor-bearing patients and animals. Sialyl-
and galactosyl-transferases have been the most extensively
studied glycosyltransferases and will be discussed independently of the other glycosyltransferases.

SIALYLTRANSFERASE

Serum sialyltransferase has been reported to be significantly elevated in several animal tumors, including rat
mammary tumors (Bosmann and Hilf, 1974; Bernaki and Kim,
1977; Evans et al., 1980), malignant melanoma (Kondo et al.,
1981), hepatomas, and leukemias (Bosmann et al., 1975).
The increase in serum sialyltransferase activity is propor-
tional to tumor size, tumor burden, and tumor age (Evans et
al., 1980; Bernaki and Kim, 1977). The source of the serum
sialyltransferase has not been determined, but it is presumed to arise from the tumor or other host tissues (Evans
et al., 1980; Bosmann et al., 1975; Kondo et al., 1981).
No studies have been reported on the serum sialyltransferase
levels in carcinogen-treated animals, although several of
the studies used transplantable tumors that were originally

chemically induced (Bernaki and Kim, 1977; Bosmann and Hilf, 1974). Sialyltransferase is measured using cytosine-5'-monophosphoryl-N-acetylneuraminic acid (CMP-NANA) radio-labeled in the sialic acid moiety and asialofetuin as the sialic acid donor and acceptor, respectively. Sialic acid incorporation into fetuin can be measured by liquid scintil-lation techniques after isolation of the protein product by high voltage paper electrophoresis, paper chromatography, or phosphotungstic acid precipitation.

Serum sialyltransferase may be a useful marker in animal tumor studies, because the high rate of false positives due to benign disease found in man can be adequately controlled. Extensive testing with known carcinogenic and noncarcino-genic compounds is needed to validate serum sialyltransfer-ase as a tumor marker in animals.

In humans, serum sialyltransferase has been found to be elevated in numerous types of tumors, including breast, colon, cervical, and testicular tumors, hepatoma, and gen-eral malignant disease (Bosmann and Hall, 1974; Dao et al., 1980; Sarjadi et al., 1980; Kessel et al., 1976; Liu et al., 1979; Ganzinger, 1977; Moser et al., 1980), while serum sialyltransferase has been reported to be lower in patients with ovarian cancer (Sarjadi et al., 1980). False negatives are reported in about 15 to 20% of people with general malignant diseases (Ganzinger, 1977; Durham et al., 1979), while the false positive rate for healthy, normal patients is 0%. The false positive rate has been reported to be as high as 100% for patients with various nonneoplas-tic diseases (Ronquist et al., 1980) including rheumatoid arthritis, liver diseases, infections (Lee et al., 1980a), hernias, inflammatory bowel disease (Ronquist et al., 1980), gastric ulcer, Parkinson's disease, heart disease, renal failure, bronchopneumonia, Crohn's disease, cholecystitis, and liver cirrhosis (Durham et al., 1979). The extensive list of benign disorders resulting in elevated serum sialyl-transferase may limit the usefulness of this enzyme as a cancer marker. A similar conclusion was reached by Weiser and Wilson (1981), who recently reviewed serum sialyltrans-ferases as tumor markers. Several of the investigators who reported high false-positive rates for serum sialyltransfer-ase used a nonquantitative assay in which either the protein substrate or CMP-NANA was limiting, which may lead to erro-neous conclusions (Ronquist et al., 1980; Durham et al., 1979). Serum sialyltransferase has been found to be a

useful prognostic tool when a malignant tumor has been diagnosed by other means (Ganzinger and Deutsch, 1980; Henderson
and Kessel, 1977; Kessel et al., 1976; Ganzinger, 1977;
Moser et al., 1980; Dao et al., 1980). Serum sialyltransferase levels have been found to depend on the tumor size
and stage of tumor growth, stage I tumors yielding lower
serum enzyme levels and stages II and III yielding increasing levels (Ganzinger, 1977; Dao et al., 1980; Ganzinger
and Deutsch, 1980). Serum levels reverted to normal with
successful therapy.

GALACTOSYLTRANSFERASE

Serum Galactosyltransferase

Total serum UDP-galactose:glycoprotein galactosyltransferase has been found to be a useful marker for ovarian
(Bhattacharya and Barlow, 1979; Bhattacharya et al., 1976;
Chatterjee et al., 1981), breast (Waalkes and Tormey, 1978;
Paone et al., 1980), pancreatic (Holyoke et al., 1979),
and lung cancer (Kijimoto-Ochiai et al., 1981) in man.
Although various other diseases (such as celiac disease,
active inflammation, active metabolic, or acute liver disease) yield higher serum galactosyltransferase elevations
compared to normal serum, statistically significant enzyme
elevations were found in the sera of patients with primary
breast carcinoma and untreated metastatic breast cancer
(Paone et al., 1980). The extent of serum enzyme elevation
was found to be related to the clinical stage of breast
cancer: significant elevations were found in 3 of 21
(14.3%) stage I, 8 of 12 (66.7%) stage II, 11 of 14 (78.6%)
stage III, and 28 of 29 (96.5%) stage IV patients. Hence,
in breast cancer, the elevation of serum galactosyltransferase corresponds with the clinical stage of disease (Paone
et al., 1980). Serum galactosyltransferase levels returned
to normal following surgical resection of tumors in 11 of
13 (84.6%) breast cancer patients. A 100% correlation of
elevated serum galactosyltransferase was found for ovarian
cancer (11 of 11) with a reduction following surgical resection of the tumor in 7 of 7 patients (Bhattacharya et al.,
1976).

Serum galactosyltransferase appears to be a good marker for
the limited tumor types investigated. A wider population of
cancer patients needs to be studied for elevation of serum
levels. A large population of normal and benign disease

controls must be evaluated to establish the false positive rate in the general population. Also, the correlation of serum enzyme elevation with the clinical stage or tumor burden needs to be evaluated to determine the limits of detection of serum galactosyltransferase.

The enzyme assay is relatively rapid, is easy to perform, requires no specialized equipment other than a scintillation counter, and should be relatively inexpensive. The assay uses asialo, agalacto-fetuin as the glycoprotein acceptor; this substrate is not yet commercially available and must be prepared from commercially available fetuin. UDP-galactose is available commercially, both cold and radiolabeled, so serum galactosyltransferase may be assayed under optimal substrate conditions. The assay of total serum galactosyl-transferase, however, cannot distinguish between the several galactosyltransferase isoenzymes found in serum. This is particularly significant, as one isoenzyme, galactosyltrans-ferase isoenzyme II, is elevated in the sera of cancer patients but is lacking in normal sera (see below).

Galactosyltransferase Isoenzyme II

Podolsky and co-workers (Podolsky et al., 1977) have demon-strated a serum galactosyltransferase isoenzyme (GT-II) in hamsters bearing polyoma-transformed BHK cells. The amount of GT-II was related to tumor growth and was detectable before tumors were visible. Normal, nontumor-bearing ani-mals had no detectable GT-II. There were no false positive or false negative results, suggesting that GT-II may be a useful cancer marker in animals.

At present, the assay of GT-II is slow, expensive, and time-consuming, requiring polyacrylamide gel electrophoresis to separate the various galactosyltransferase isoenzymes before enzyme analysis. Recently, Podolsky and Weiser (1979) puri-fied human serum GT-II to homogeneity and demonstrated that it is structurally and kinetically distinct from the galac-tosyltransferase found in normal serum. This finding should stimulate the development of a very sensitive immunodiag-nostic assay for GT-II, resulting in a rapid, simple, and inexpensive assay to be used in the wider evaluation of GT-II as a cancer marker. The studies need to be extended to other animal species, other tumors systems, and chemically induced tumors. GT-II is a promising tumor marker for use both in animals and in humans. Weiser and Wilson (1981) reached a similar conclusion concerning the use of GT-II.

Podolsky and co-workers have characterized a UDP-galactose: glycoprotein galactosyltransferase isoenzyme that is not found in normal human sera but is found in the serum of cancer patients (Podolsky and Weiser, 1975; Weiser et al., 1976; Podolsky et al., 1978; Podolsky and Weiser, 1979; Podolsky et al., 1981). Serum galactosyltransferase isoenzyme II (GT-II) was found in 43 of 58 (74%) carcinoma patients, whereas only 2 of 39 (5%) controls exhibited detectable GT-II (Podolsky et al., 1979). Further examination of false-positive results in patients showed that 3 of 15 (20%) with severe alcoholic hepatitis and 18 of 20 (90%) patients with severe celiac disease had detectable GT-II. GT-II has been specifically associated with pancreatic (Podolsky et al., 1981), colonic (Whitehead et al., 1979), colorectal, gastrointestinal (Podolsky et al., 1978), and ovarian (Chatterjee et al., 1979) cancer; hepatomas (Waxman et al., 1980); and bronchogenic carcinomas (Weiser et al., 1976; Podolsky et al., 1978; Moser et al., 1980; Pohl and Moser, 1978; Yogeeswaran, 1980).

Although extensive studies specifically correlating GT-II with cancer in general have not been performed, GT-II has been found to be one of the best markers for pancreatic cancer so far studied. A false-positive rate of only 1.4% for benign pancreatic disease and 4.4% for acute or chronic pancreatitis, coupled with a false-negative rate of 32.8%, results in a specificity rating of 98.3% for GT-II in pancreatic cancer (Podolsky et al., 1981). Considering the low false-positive rates for GT-II, and relatively high association with cancer (approximately 70%, Podolsky et al., 1978), it would seem judicious to examine the statistical usefulness of this enzyme marker in other cancer types. Studies that need to be performed include determinations of: (1) minimum detectable tumor burden, (2) GT-II levels and clinical stage of cancer, (3) association with benign disease, and (4) usefulness of GT-II in conjunction with other tumor markers for more accurate diagnosis.

OTHER GLYCOSYLTRANSFERASES

There are several reports of alterations of glycosyltransferases (other than the sialyl- and galactosyltransferases) associated with cancer. These include fucosyltransferase (Kessel et al., 1979; Kuzmits et al., 1979; Kuhns and Schoentag, 1981), N-acetylgalactosaminyltransferase (Kuhns and Schoentag, 1981; Kim and Isaacs, 1975; Chatterjee et al., 1979), and N-acetylglucosaminyltransferase (Kim and

Isaacs, 1975; Chatterjee et al., 1979). To date, the reports in the literature are insufficient for evaluation of the usefulness of these glycosyltransferases as cancer markers.

VII

Glycosidases and Blood Carbohydrates

A.E. Brandt

A.E. Brandt

β–GLUCURONIDASE

β–Glucuronidase is of interest as a possible tumor marker because of its role in breaking down extracellular matrix glycosaminoglycan structures. The breakdown of the extra-cellular matrix facilitates both the escape of metastatic tumor cells from the primary tumor site and the establish-ment of secondary tumors. In animals, β–glucuronidase studies have been limited primarily to whole tissue, whereas in humans, blood and cerebrospinal fluid have been analyzed. Increased β–glucuronidase levels in the cerebrospinal fluid have been correlated with several specific central nervous system tumors.

Rats (Brown, 1978; Kitagawa, 1976; Harris et al., 1977), hamsters (Ismail et al., 1978), mice (Laurent et al., 1977), and dogs (Hagerstrand, 1973) have been used in determining the association between β–glucuronidase and tumors. Azoxy-methane (Brown, 1978), N-2-fluorenyl-acetamide (Kitagawa, 1976), and $[^{32}P]$ (Harris et al., 1977) have been used to induce tumors of the colon, liver, and bone, respectively, in rats, while diethylstilbestrol was used to induce renal tumors in hamsters (Ismail, 1978). The tumor tissue in each case was examined histologically for increased β–glucuronid-ase and compared to control tissue. In no cases were body fluids (blood, urine, or cerebrospinal fluid) assayed for enzyme activity. In general, an increase in β–glucuronidase activity detected by histologic (qualitative) methods was observed in association with the tumor tissue. Therefore β-glucuronidase may be of interest as a potential tumor marker in experimental animals. It should be noted that β-glucuronidase levels have been observed to vary between strains of the same animal species, especially rats, mice, and hamsters (Ballantyne and Bright, 1978; Chang et al., 1968; Tamura and Matsumoto, 1980). Further evaluation, however, is needed to assess this enzyme. Future research should include:

(1) Quantitative evaluation of enzyme activity in accessible biological fluids.

(2) Tumor types that give rise to increased β-glucuronidase.

(3) Benign states that may give rise to increased enzyme levels (such as drug metabolism studies).

(4) Minimum tumor burden giving rise to increased β-glucuronidase levels.

In humans β-glucuronidase seems to be of little use in the early detection of tumors. The elevation of this enzyme in serum is quite variable and probably depends on the tumor burden and clinical state. β-Glucuronidase has been most useful in the detection, diagnosis, and prognosis of several CNS tumors, including neoplastic meningitis and meningeal lymphoma (Schold et al., 1980; Shuttleworth et al., 1980). Various other CNS diseases, such as tuberculous and other bacterial meningitides, can also cause elevated levels of β-glucuronidase in the cerebral spinal fluid, suggesting that other tools are required to confirm the diagnosis.

The assay of β-glucuronidase in biological fluids is simple and very sensitive. A routine fluorimetric method using umbelliferal-β-glucuronide as the substrate is available commercially and could be readily applied to fluids obtained from animals. There may be difficulty, however, in obtaining cerebral spinal fluid from small laboratory animals. For β-glucuronidase to become a useful tumor marker, nonneoplastic disease controls must be evaluated more extensively.

SIALIC ACID

Tumor cells possess an increased net negative surface charge due to increased amounts of sialic acid on cell-surface glycoproteins and glycolipids. With tumor growth, some of these cell-surface sialic-acid-containing glycoproteins and glycolipids are shed into the circulation and result

in increased serum sialic acid levels. This increase has
been found in animals and in man, but only when the tumor
burden has become quite large. Sialic acid may be a useful
tumor marker for the diagnosis and prognosis of tumors in
animals and in man. Yogeeswaran (1980) recently reviewed
the association between sialic acid and tumors.

Experimental tumors in rats (Bernacki and Kim, 1977; Kloppel
and Morre, 1980) and mice (Khadapkar et al., 1975) show
increased tumor-associated sialic acid. When transplantable
hepatomas induced with N-2-fluorenylacetamide were examined
(Kloppel and Morre, 1980), higher sialic acid levels were
associated with the tumors than with untreated liver. Non-
metastatic tumor lines showed lower N-acetylneuraminic acid-
galactose-glucose-N-acetylsphingosine (GM_3) and a higher
ratio of total monosialogangliosides to disialogangliosides
than did metastatic lines. Ganglioside patterns of metastatic lines closely resembled the ganglioside pattern of
normal liver. The changes in tissue and serum ganglioside
sialic acid were consistent features of liver tumorigenesis following N-2-fluoroenylacetamide administration and
appeared to be early events not directly related to tumor
cell differentiation or metastasis. Tumor-cell-surface
glycoproteins were not evaluated.

Bernacki and Kim (1977) found an increase in serum protein-
bound sialic acid in metastasizing mammary tumors transplanted in rats and believed it to be derived from the
shedding of tumor-cell-surface glycoproteins. They suggested that the presence of tumor cell surface glycoproteins
in the serum may help the tumor cell escape from the immune
system of the host and thus to play a role in tumor metastasis. Khadapkar et al. (1975) suggest that the increased
serum sialic acid associated with tumorigenesis may be a
general characteristic of proliferative cell growth and
thus not unique to tumorigenesis.

Total serum sialic acid can be quantitated following mild
acid hydrolysis by the thiobarbituric acid assay developed
by Warren (1959) or the recently developed, more sensitive
fluorimetric thiobarbituric acid assay (Hammond and Papermaster, 1976). A rapid, high-performance liquid chromatography (HPLC) assay for sialic acid has recently been
introduced (Silver et al., 1981).

The serum sialic acid level may possibly serve as an
early marker for tumorigenesis in animals. However,

only preliminary studies on its applicability have been
performed, and there are insufficient data at this time for
statistical analysis. The following determinations need to
be made:

- Serum sialic acid levels following administration
  of known carcinogens.

- Minimum detectable tumor burden.

- The source of increased serum sialic acid (tumor
  versus host organs, e.g., liver).

- The specificity of serum sialic acid for tumors
  versus benign diseases such as liver toxicity and
  disease, inflammation, and viral infection.

In man, serum sialic acid levels have been found to increase
in cancer. Waalkes et al. (1978) found that occult metastases of breast cancer could be detected two to four months
earlier when serum sialic acid levels were evaluated than
when conventional laboratory techniques were used. In contrast, Hogan-Ryan et al. (1980) found that increased serum
sialic acid levels were associated only with advanced (stage
IV) breast cancer. Increased serum sialic acid levels have
also been associated with malignant melanoma (Silver et al.,
1980) and bronchogenic carcinoma (Coombes et al., 1978),
and altered sialomucins have been associated with colorectal
cancers.

The assays for serum sialic acid are the same as those
described for animals. Serum sialic acid levels seem to be
useful in the diagnosis of cancer in man and may provide a
prognostic indicator for the effectiveness of therapeutic
regimens. However, studies relating to the minimum detectable tumor burden, nononcogenic disease controls as a source
of false positives (liver disease, inflammation, infection,
respiratory disease, arthritis), association with type of
tumor, and application to larger patient populations for
statistical analysis need to be undertaken before serum
sialic acid levels can be judged as a reliable tumor marker.

FUCOSE

Serum protein-bound fucose levels and changes in the fucose
content of tumors have not been evaluated in experimental
animals.

In man, serum protein-bound fucose has been found to be increased in metastatic breast cancer (22 of 29, 76%) (Mrochek et al., 1975; Mrochek et al., 1976; Solanki et al., 1978; Waalkes et al., 1978) as well as in pancreatic, stomach, urinary bladder, kidney, and lung cancer (Pradhan et al., 1979). A relatively easy colorimetric assay for fucose is available as well as a sensitive HPLC assay. Gas chromatography (GC) has not been applied to the analysis of serum protein-bound fucose levels, but GC assays should be more rapid and sensitive than current HPLC and colorimetric assays. The applicability of serum protein-bound fucose as a tumor marker in animals needs to be established. In man, other diseases that could lead to increased fucose levels needs to be examined and evaluated. Further testing of the specificity of fucose levels for various types of cancer, and an increased tumor population base for better statistical analysis, are also recommended.

GLYCOSIDASE AND BLOOD CARBOHYDRATE MARKERS

Table VII-1 shows the glycosidases and blood carbohydrates deemed to be unlikely cancer markers at this time in animal screens, along with those for which there was insufficient information by which to evaluate their potential, and the reasons for their tentative dispositions.

Table VII-1

GLYCOSIDASES AND BLOOD CARBOHYDRATES FOR WHICH
THERE WAS NOT ENOUGH INFORMATION TO EVALUATE POTENTIAL

Compound	Comment	References
Unlikely Markers		
Inter-α-trypsin inhibitor	Normal serum component	Chawla et al., 1978
Serum protein-bound mannose	No significant elevation	Mrochek et al., 1976
Serum protein-bound galactose	No significant elevation	Mrochek et al., 1976
General serum carbohydrate levels	Only sialic acid, fucose may be of interest	Mrochek et al., 1976; Waalkes et al., 1978
Lectins	Useful only as a research tool for characterizing cell surface carbohydrate structures	Nicolson, 1980

(Continued)

Table VII-1 (Concluded)

Compound	Comment	References
β-Glucosidase	Not elevated	Klohs et al., 1981; Bosmann et al., 1975
α-Mannosidase	No difference between normal and malignant tissue	Bosmann et al., 1975 Klohs et al., 1981
β-Galactosidase	Not elevated	Bosmann et al., 1975
α-Fucosidase	Not elevated	Bosmann et al., 1975
Potential Markers		
β-N-Acetyl-glucosaminidase	Found secreted into culture media of rat osteosarcoma cells	Harris et al., 1977
Neuraminidase	Assayed in tumor tissue homogenates	Bosmann and Hall, 1974

VIII

Carbohydrate Metabolizing Enzymes

R.H. Suva, C.A. Tyson

INTRODUCTION

The observation that cancer cells have an increased rate
of respiration suggests that enzymes active in carbohydrate
catabolism and energy generation might be altered in the
malignant state. However, most of these enzymes do not
appear to be useful as serum markers for the early detection of cancer in animals. Most changes in enzyme level or
isozyme pattern occur in the cancerous tissue and are seen
in serum only in advanced disease, if at all. Two enzymes
that appear to be exceptions are lactate dehydrogenase and
fructose diphosphate aldolase; these are discussed below.

LACTATE DEHYDROGENASE

Animal Studies

Lactate dehydrogenase (LDH) catalyzes the conversion of
L-lactate to L-pyruvate in mammalian cells. The enzyme is
broadly distributed, and quantitative assessments in sera,
while indicative of cell necrosis and other lesions, are
not organ-specific (Tietz, 1976). Nevertheless, serum LDH
is a convenient and inexpensive parameter to measure, and
anomalous results can be investigated by histopathologic
techniques or isozyme analysis in animal studies. Therefore, despite its nonspecificity, its usefulness as a preneoplastic marker is worth consideration; in fact, its wide
tissue distribution might be advantageous as a general
marker to complement others.

Studies that might provide data to assess LDH's value for this purpose in animal assays are few. Nievel et al. (1976) and Tyndall et al. (1978) found that neither circulatory nor tissue LDH was necessarily correlated with or sensitive to liver damage and hepatocellular carcinomas in rats or mice given various carcinogens and noncarcinogens daily for up to three months.

Isozyme analysis may be more useful when analyzed as they were in hexachlorocyclohexane feeding studies in mice. The liver enzyme patterns showed a decrease in the faster-moving LDH-1 and LDH-2 bands at sacrifice after two months when compared with control LDH bands (Thakore et al., 1981). Concomitant with these changes, a new protein, presumably α-fetoprotein, based on its electrophoretic mobility, appeared in the serum of the treated animals. Tumors did not develop in them for six months, by which time the new LDH bands had almost disappeared (Thakore et al., 1981). In another study, single injections of each of six different carcinogens in weanling mice (in a lung tumor bioassay) elevated lung glycolytic enzymes 28 days later. Total LDH activity increased by about 50% and the LDH H and M subunit ratio was significantly decreased; eight noncarcinogens tested under the same conditions failed to produce these changes (Rady et al., 1980). The test concentrations of all chemicals were near the maximal tolerated doses, and the changes observed were characteristic of those involved in tissue regeneration. They appeared to be more extensive in the animals exposed to carcinogens. The isozyme pattern in affected mouse lungs resembled that in normal fetal lung and in lungs with pulmonary adenomas that form later (Rady et al., 1979). Whether these same patterns appear during lung regeneration following exposure to nononcogenic toxins needs to be resolved.

Serum LDH-1, associated with human endodermal sinus tumors transplanted to nude mice, continued to serve as a useful marker for tumor growth, along with α-fetoprotein (Takeuchi et al., 1979). In contrast to the feeding study with hexachlorocyclohexane (Thakore et al., 1981), however, the LDH-1 band was elevated. With the hamster cheek-pouch model for squamous cell carcinoma, alterations in LDH were not seen histochemically until malignancy developed, but succinate and glucose-6-phosphate dehydrogenases became elevated much earlier and reverted to near-normal levels when true neoplastic lesions became established (Evans et al., 1980a).

None of these changes were found with benign hyperplastic lesions.

This review of the more recent literature and other published reviews do not provide enough data with which to assess LDH's potential value, but the little information available on quantitative determinations of total serum LDH is not encouraging. A major reason is that chronic respiratory diseases common in rats and blood hemolysis during sampling can cause high and variable background levels, compromising the value of quantitative LDH analysis in serum. The studies with mice cited above, however, suggest that isozyme analysis may presage tumor formation before it appears. LDH isozyme analysis of selected major organ tissues and blood during or after subchronic studies in this species deserves further consideration.

Human Studies

LDH has received considerable attention in man, and its potential diagnostic value has been examined for many types of cancer including those of the central nervous system (CNS), ovarian, cervical, testicular, vesicular (urinary bladder), prostatic, renal, hepatic, uterine, mammary, and gastrointestinal tumors, and leukemia (Lee et al., 1980c; Motomiya et al., 1975; Posey et al., 1979). It has also been measured in cerebrospinal fluid (CSF), serum, and urine.

As with several other enzyme indicators of CNS tumors, evaluations of the usefulness of LDH were not generally encouraging (Hildebrand, 1973; Seidenfeld and Marton, 1978, 1979; Wasserstrom et al., 1981). In one study, low-grade malignancies and benign tumors could not be distinguished by LDH levels in cyst fluid (Pullicino et al., 1979). The levels of LDH and other markers were enhanced with advanced malignancies, but the association of these changes with the tumors was complicated by the presence of edema. In 1978, a review of biochemical markers for CNS tumors indicated that analyzing LDH in CSF was not useful for screening and was not as predictive or efficient as analyzing for aldolase and desmosterol (Seidenfeld and Marton, 1978). A more recent review noted that the predominance of bands 1 and 2 over bands 5 and 4 in CSF shifted with neoplastic disease, but the change apparently was not specific and information in the literature was conflicting (Wasserstrom et al., 1981). Lack of both tumor specificity and sensitivity were also noted by other reviewers (Seidenfeld and Marton, 1979).

(CSF could not be monitored readily in routine animal studies because brain tumors in animals exposed to environmental chemicals occur too rarely to warrant the added expense of collecting and analyzing this fluid for early indications of tumorigenesis.)

Early reports suggested that urinary LDH might be a highly useful indicator for renal and bladder cancer, usually in conjunction with other indicators such as alkaline phosphatase (ALP), but its lack of specificity for malignancies (Amador et al., 1963; Dorfman et al., 1963a, 1963b; Boettiger et al., 1966) limits its usefulness for detecting renal carcinoma (Hautmann, 1979). There is a notable lack of correlation between changes in serum and urinary LDH activity because urinary LDH is related only to disease of the upper urinary tract (Dorfman et al., 1963b), whereas serum LDH can relate to bladder carcinoma as well (Amador et al., 1963). LDH content is high in bladder carcinomas (Kawamura, 1980), and Amador et al. (1963) recommended earlier that both LDH and alkaline phosphatase be monitored for the routine diagnosis of renal adenocarcinomas. Isozyme analysis was useful in sharpening the diagnosis of bladder tumors (Motomiya et al., 1975). The LDH-5 to LDH-1 ratio in urine was significantly elevated in the majority of patients, and the LDH-5 band was shown to originate from the tumors themselves. Serum LDH was also one of the most sensitive indicators among several evaluated for prostatic cancer, but the latent nature of the disease, in which clinical manifestations are too seldom apparent, makes decisions regarding its practicality for early detection of the disease difficult (Catalona and Menon, 1981).

Although using LDH for detecting testicular tumors is controversial rather than promising (Uchijima et al., 1979), some clinicians still prefer to use it in conjunction with other markers for managing treatment of such tumors (Bosl et al., 1981). Similarly, LDH by itself is not sensitive for detecting ovarian carcinomas (Burrows, 1980), but LDH combined with RNase was one of the better marker systems for distinguishing between benign and malignant ovarian tumors (Dobryszycka et al., 1979). LDH combined with other markers could detect cervical carcinomas (Sarjadi et al., 1980) and LDH combined with GGT could detect hepatic metastases in gastrointestinal cancer (Huguier and Lacaine, 1981).

One area that has not received sufficient attention is the use of isozyme analysis to increase the sensitivity of the

LDH indicator for early diagnosis of cancers. Recently, Anderson and Kovacik (1981) reported an unusual isozyme of LDH in cells transformed by the Kirsten murine sarcoma virus. The isozyme appears to be present at much higher levels (as much as 10 to 100 times higher) than in normal tissues in a variety of human carcinomas compared with other LDH isozymes. Shifts in the isozyme patterns of a number of enzymes including LDH have also been reported to occur in malignant tissue from uterine cancer (Marshall et al., 1979). If marker isozymes of LDH can be found to occur early in sera, they might be useful as general diagnostic indicators for malignancies. The existence of counterpart isozymes might be similarly useful in animal studies for screening for carcinogenicity.

FRUCTOSE DIPHOSPHATE ALDOLASE

Fructose diphosphate (FDP) aldolase cleaves FDP to glyceraldehyde phosphate and dihydroxyacetone phosphate. Although we found no studies of this enzyme as a cancer marker in animals, recent work in humans suggests that this enzyme has broad potential. The level of FDP aldolase does not dramatically change in humans with cancer (Dacha, 1980), but some studies indicate that the isozyme pattern can provide useful information.

In one study the muscle isozyme of FDP aldolase was measured by radioimmunoassay in sera from cancer patients, and found to be higher in 86 of 129 patients (Asaka, 1979; Asaka et al., 1980). The only other disease with an elevated isozyme level was progressive muscular dystrophy. A number of different tumors elevated the marker, including hepatic, pancreatic, gastric, pulmonary, lymphoid, and colorectal, as did leukemia, also. Unfortunately, the clinical stage of cancer in these patients was not described. Further work is needed to determine whether the isozyme is elevated in serum from tumor-bearing animals and whether the elevation occurs early enough to be useful.

In a similar study, the brain isozyme was measured in CSF from patients with CNS tumors (reviewed by Seidenfeld and Marton, 1978, 1979) and was found to be elevated in 21 of 39 patients with CNS tumors, compared to four of 67 controls. Thus, the marker has a low sensitivity, but a relatively high level of specificity. Again, the utility of this marker for the early detection of cancer in animals cannot be assessed from these studies. Although it is probably impractical to sample CSF from small animals at this time, these results and those presented above indicate that it may be worthwhile to examine the FDP aldolase iso-zyme pattern in animals exposed to carcinogens.

OTHER CARBOHYDRATE METABOLIZING ENZYMES

A large number of related enzymes have been examined for their potential as cancer markers. In general, they have been studied in humans only, and to a limited extent. Their potential utility in animal carcinogenesis screening systems has not been evaluated. Table VIII-1 lists these markers, along with their reasons for being included in this category.

Table VIII-1

ENZYMES JUDGED TO HAVE LIMITED OR UNKNOWN POTENTIAL
FOR THE EARLY DETECTION OF CANCER IN ANIMALS

Enzyme	Comment(s)	Reference(s)
Hexosaminidase	Enzyme found only in cells	Brattain et al., 1979 Sakamoto et al., 1979
Isocitrate dehydrogenase	Enzyme studied only in cells or CSF; latter fluid inaccessible in animals	Dutu et al., 1980; Nievel et al., 1976; Seidenfeld and Marton, 1978; Wasserstrom et al., 1981
Malate dehydrogenase	Enzyme lower in tumor	Stocco and Hutson, 1980
Malic enzyme	No data correlating with cancer	Curtin and Snell, 1980
Succinate dehydrogenase	Enzyme only in cells; activity decreases in tumors	Dutu et al., 1980; Evans et al., 1980a; Hagerstrand, 1973; Lipsky et al., 1981
Lysozyme	Studied in CSF; low predictive value	Coombes et al., 1977; Seidenfeld and Marton, 1978; Wasserstrom et al., 1981

(Continued)

Table VIII-1 (Continued)

Enzyme	Comment(s)	Reference(s)
Sucrase, Trehalase	Nonspecific; only in cells	Matsukura et al., 1979
β-Galactosidase	No correlation with cancer	Dolbeare et al., 1980
Hexokinase	Changes are small and unpredictable	Curtin and Snell, 1980; Dacha et al., 1980; Herzfeld and Greengard, 1980; Herzfeld et al., 1980; Marshall et al., 1979; Rady et al., 1979,1980
Glucokinase	Changes small and unpredictable	Curtin and Snell, 1980
Phosphohexose isomerase	No correlation with cancer	Dacha et al., 1980; DeYoung et al., 1980; Pullicino et al., 1979; Seidenfeld and Marton, 1978
PEP Carboxykinase	Changes small	Curtin and Snell, 1980

(Continued)

Table VIII-1 (Continued)

Enzyme	Comment(s)	Reference(s)
Pyruvate kinase	Changes small	Dacha et al., 1980
Phosphoglucomutase	No correlation with cancer	Dacha et al., 1980
Lipoamide dehydrogenase	Marker lower in cancer	Marshall et al., 1979; Stocco and Hutson, 1980
Transketolase	No data correlating with cancer	Dacha et al., 1980
6-Phosphogluconate dehydrogenase	No correlation with cancer	Asanami, 1979; Dacha et al., 1980; Dutu et al., 1980; Fischer and Grund, 1979; Marshall et al., 1979
Glucose-6-phosphate dehydrogenase	Serum changes are small and unpredictable; the only significant changes in activity occur within cancer-ous cells	Asanami, 1979; Curtin and Snell, 1980; Dacha et al., 1980; Du et al., 1979; Dutu et al., 1980; Evans et al., 1980a; Fischer and Grund, 1979;

(Continued)

Table VIII-1 (Concluded)

Enzyme	Comment(s)	Reference(s)
Phosphofructo-kinase	No significant serum changes	Herzfeld and Greengard, 1980; Herzfeld et al., 1980; Lipsky et al., 1981; Nievel et al., 1976
Glucose phosphate isomerase	Changes small; studied in CSF only	Dacha et al., 1980; Rady et al., 1979, 1980 Seidenfeld and Marton, 1979; Wasserstrom et al., 1981

IX

Other Enzyme Markers

R.A. Howd

ACID PHOSPHATASE

Acid phosphatase (AP) was one of the first substances evaluated as a potential tumor marker, and there is consequently a large and diverse literature on its use in the detection of cancer in humans. This lysosomal enzyme is found in virtually all types of cells, with different isoenzyme forms in many tissues. AP can be released from cells due to tissue cytolysis or other damage, including that associated with tumor growth.

AP has most commonly been evaluated as a marker for tumors of the prostate gland. It has shown promise because of the relatively high concentration of AP in the human prostate and the resulting large, but variable, increases in its serum level caused by prostatic disease (Schwartz, 1978; Chu et al., 1980; Jacobi, 1979; Rustin, 1980; Beckley et al., 1980).

There is little reason to think that AP might be a practical diagnostic marker for the chemical induction of tumors in animals, including those of the prostate. Prostatic tumors have a low incidence in laboratory species, and there is no good animal model for evaluating their induction (Claflin et al., 1980; Coffey and Isaacs, 1980). In addition, the prostate glands of the common laboratory animal species have much lower AP levels than do those of humans (i.e, dog 5%, rat 0.08% of human concentrations), so the release of this enzyme into the circulation by prostatic tumors would result in relatively small elevations of serum levels. Thus, a

very sensitive and specific radioimmunoassay for prostatic
AP would be required. Development of a reliable assay has
been a continuing problem for human studies (Chu et al.,
1978; Belville et al., 1979; Jacobi, 1979; Beckley et al.,
1980; Farnsworth et al., 1980; Vihko et al., 1980; Grayhack
et al., 1980; Zweig and Van Steirteghem, 1981), and new
assays are required for the immunologically distinct animal
isozyme(s) (Lee et al., 1980). As in humans, animal prostatic tumors may vary considerably in their AP content
(Drago et al., 1980), so a similarly high (40 to 60%) false-
negative rate might be expected.

Early human studies demonstrated a positive correlation of
serum AP levels with prostatic cancer, but rather poor specificity, using a biochemical assay of total AP activities.
Later work has generally used more sensitive immunologic
methods specific for the prostatic isozyme, but with little
improvement in the results (Beckley et al., 1980; Farnsworth
et al., 1980). The general conclusion among clinicians has
been that the low predictive value of AP measurements makes
them of little use in the diagnosis of prostatic cancer,
but that repeated AP measurements may be useful in evaluating the prognosis for specific individuals with confirmed
prostate cancer (Tormey et al., 1979; Kiesling and Watson,
1980; Watson and Tang, 1980; Torti and Carter, 1980).

Measurement of serum AP would not be expected to be valuable
in the diagnosis of cancers of other tissues, such as the
ovary (Dobryszycka et al., 1979), because of the relatively
modest increase in serum levels and the possibility of false
positives due to nonspecific tissue damage. Neither does
measuring AP in tissues appear to be of much value in cancer
studies (Hagerstrand, 1973; Bosmann and Hall, 1974; Nievel
et al., 1976; Davey et al., 1977; Tatematsu et al., 1977;
Ismail et al., 1978; Lisiewicz et al., 1978; Ikegwuonu et
al., 1980; Beckley et al., 1980; Fischer and Gevers, 1980;
Micheau et al., 1980; Rustin, 1980; Catovsky et al., 1981;
Uchida et al., 1981), except in the diagnosis of prostatic
metastases, in which an abnormal level of prostate-specific
enzyme may be found by biopsy (Belville et al., 1979; Heaney
et al., 1981). Excess AP may be found in the cerebrospinal
fluid (CSF) of people with brain tumors, but many other
enzymes are also commonly elevated, and AP may be less specific as a CSF tumor marker than other enzymes (Wasserstrom
et al., 1981).

The diagnosis of preneoplastic lesions in tissues by analyzing AP levels is also not promising, because AP tissue levels may go up, go down, or stay the same after animals are treated with cancer-inducing chemicals (Nievel et al., 1976; Tatematsu et al., 1977; Ismail et al., 1978; Ikegwuono et al., 1980).

Because of the considerable attention being devoted to animal models for the study of prostatic tumors (Murphy, 1980), specific animal prostate AP assays may be developed shortly. However, as detailed above, the possibility that AP analysis would be useful in the general screening for carcinogenic chemicals in animals seems remote.

CATHEPSINS

Cathepsins are a family of lysosomal proteinases found in most tissues of humans and experimental animals. Cathepsins might be expected to be released in relatively large amounts (along with other lysosomal enzymes) from growing tumors or adjacent tissues because of the high metabolic and cytolytic activities in such tissues. In a few studies these proteinases have been evaluated as cancer markers in humans, but not in animals, except *in vitro,* where cathepsins were not promising as a cytologic marker of transformation of cells (Dolbeare et al., 1980). Specific cathepsin isozymes might be useful as serum markers for cancer in different tissues, but the isozyme pattern probably varies across species, so data from human studies are not directly applicable to animals.

The blood level of cathepsin B1 was specifically and greatly increased (compared with several other lysosomal enzymes) in women after prenatal diethylstilbestrol (DES) exposure, and was correlated with the degree of aberration in vaginal pathology (Pietras et al., 1978). Such a correlation with a specific lesion induced by a given drug or drug class may indicate that assay of cathepsin(s) could be of value in analogous animal tests should there be a relevant animal model for this estrogen effect.

In a study of serum enzymes in women with ovarian tumors, cathepsin was shown to be less valuable as a marker of tumor burden than ribonuclease in combination with amino transferases and lactate dehydrogenase (Dobryszycka et al., 1979).

While tumors other than those induced by DES in the vagina can clearly release high levels of cathepsins (Poole et al., 1978), the extent to which increased serum cathepsin(s) might be correlated with body burden of various tumor types is unknown.

We would regard this as a marker of low priority for further study, except for one report (Pietras et al., 1978) that indicated its utility in a well-described type of human chemical carcinogenesis. In such a specific context, assay of cathepsin(s) may have value in animal testing. Sensitive radioimmunoassays for animal tissue isozymes will probably be required for suitable results.

AMYLASE

Serum amylases can be derived from several different tissues, but the major circulating forms are apparently from the parotid gland or pancreas (Takeuchi et al., 1975). Pancreatic tumors can release high levels of amylase (Rao et al., 1980), but increased serum levels in pancreatic cancer in humans have not been well documented (Holyoke et al., 1979). At this time we have no information on the applicability of using serum amylase levels as a marker for pancreatic or parotid cancer (or cancer at other sites) in experimental animals, but because of the relatively recent development of suitable models of pancreatic cancer in animals, such information may be available soon (see Oncology Overview--Selected Abstracts on Pancreatic Carcinogenesis, USDHEW, 1980).

CREATINE KINASE BB

Creatine kinase BB has been described as a tumor marker in various human cancers (Van Steirteghem and Zweig, 1981) and compared with prostatic acid phosphatase in serum. No recent animal studies were found.

NEURON-SPECIFIC ENOLASE

Neuron-specific enolase (NSE) is a glycolytic enzyme that has been immunocytochemically detected as early as the ninth embryonic day in the ventral horn motor neurons and dorsal root ganglion of the quail (Maxwell, 1982). In rat cell embryonic culture, a dramatic rise of the isoenzyme from

13 to 24 days in differentiating neuronal cells was demonstrated, whereas glial, ependymal, and neuroblastic cells remained unstained.

In 94 newly diagnosed patients with small-cell lung cancer, serum NSE was raised above 12.0 ng/ml in 39% of those having a limited stage of disease. Levels correlated with response to therapy (Carney et al., 1982). The tumors were thought to be APUD in type. Information is inadequate to assess the applicability of NSE for an animal tumor marker.

MISCELLANEOUS ENZYME MARKERS

Many other enzymes have been evaluated as potential markers for cancer, either in body fluids or in tumors or tumor exudates. Acylase (Warwas et al., 1977) and hemopexin (Hagerstrand, 1973) did not give promising results when evaluated as markers in human sera. Histaminase has been reported to be elevated in serum from thyroid cancer patients (Schwartz, 1978) and in exudates from many tumors (Lin et al., 1979), but the data are inconclusive about whether it might have utility as a circulating cancer marker.

In tumors, enzymes that have been reported to be elevated include peptidyl proline hydroxylase (Herzfeld et al., 1980; Herzfeld and Greengard, 1980), esterases (Schwartz, 1976; Micheau et al., 1980), protease (Bosmann and Hall, 1974), and diamine oxidase (Sessa et al., 1981). Such findings do not indicate that serum levels of the enzymes might be elevated also, because tumor concentrations of other potential markers are not well correlated with their serum levels (Davey et al., 1977; Tatematsu et al., 1977; Ikegwuonu et al., 1980; Uchida et al., 1981). Thus, there is no evidence that the above enzymes might have potential as markers in body fluids, although they may deserve further consideration as cytologic markers.

X

Glycoproteins and Glycolipids

A.E. Brandt

INTRODUCTION

Numerous glycoproteins and glycolipids have been found useful as markers in the diagnosis and prognosis of tumors in
humans. However, except where noted, very few or no studies
have been performed in vivo in animal systems. Emphasis has
tended to be on mechanisms of tumorigenesis (e.g., fibronectin) rather than on cancer detection. Research directed
toward using glycoproteins and glycolipids as markers for
the early detection of cancer in animals is lacking and suggests an area for future research if such markers are to be
used in carcinogenesis screening in animals. Markers that
have been or, with further development, may prove to be useful in humans and/or animals are discussed below.

FIBRONECTIN

Fibronectin is a cell-surface-adhesive glycoprotein found
in reduced amounts on tumor cell surfaces. It is also a
normal serum component (cold insoluble globulin). The
papers reviewed produced suggestive evidence of its utility
as a marker. Catalona and Menon (1981) reported that fibronectin had a 42% sensitivity and a 97% specificity for human
prostatic cancer. Animal studies have been concerned mainly
with fibronectin on tumor cell surfaces, with little emphasis on serum levels. The animal results suggest that fibronectin could be a useful marker if background studies were
performed relating fibronectin levels to carcinogen doses,

extent of tumor burden, and other diseases. A rapid, sensitive radioimmunoassay is available for fibronectin.

FETAL SULFOGLYCOPROTEIN ANTIGEN

Fetal sulfoglycoprotein antigen (FSA) has been used for the diagnosis of gastric carcinoma in man (Rennert, 1978; Tormey et al., 1979; Hakkinen et al., 1980). Approximately 90% of gastric carcinoma patients are reported to show elevated FSA (Rennert, 1978; Tormey et al., 1979), while the incidence in the general population is low (approximately 1% in a survey of 14,000 individuals; Rennert, 1978). In a Finnish mass screening of 39,659 individuals, 3,508 individuals (8.8%) were found to be FSA positive. In these 3,508 FSA-positive individuals, 36 gastric carcinomas, one gastric carcinoid, and 10 tubular adenomas were detected. The author did not discuss the reasons for the high number of false-positive results, but gastric ulcers and chronic infections that are therapy-resistant and cause the expression of embryonic antigens (Rennert, 1978) may be the source. Detecting FSA is by radioimmunoassay, so it should be rapid, sensitive, inexpensive, and require only a centrifuge and gamma counter as major equipment. The assay is performed on gastric juice secretions, so sampling requires patient compliance. In general, FSA seems to be a good marker for gastric carcinoma in man. No animal studies have been reported, but the large number of drugs that cause cancer of the gastrointestinal tract in animals should make it worth developing.

α_1-ACID GLYCOPROTEIN

By itself, α_1-acid glycoprotein has not proven to be a useful cancer marker. However, in conjunction with α_1-antitrypsin, it was found to be effective in differentiating between malignant hepatocellular carcinoma and the benign liver diseases, cirrhosis and hepatitis (Chio and Oon, 1979). Hollinshead and Chuang (1978) found that the α_1-acid glycoprotein:prealbumin ratio was markedly higher in patients with early lung cancer (4.17), late lung cancer (8.78), bladder cancer (8.92), colon cancer (13.77), and melanoma (9.22) than in normal people (0.79), heavy smokers (1.24), or patients with nononcogenic diseases (1.67). The α_1-acid glycoprotein:prealbumin ratio for people with breast cancer was 2.43, suggesting that α_1-acid glycoprotein is not a marker for breast cancer, which agrees with other studies

(Cowen et al., 1978; Coombes et al., 1977; Coombes et al., 1980). Antibodies directed against α_1-acid glycoprotein are available, which should enable a rapid, sensitive radio-immunoassay. No animal studies relating α_1-acid glycoprotein to cancer have been reported.

α_1-ANTITRYPSIN

α_1-Antitrypsin is an endogenous serum component that inhibits trypsin-like proteases. Patients who are genetically deficient in α_1-antitrypsin are predisposed to emphysema and possibly to additional protease-induced disease states. Some cancer patients show elevated α_1-antitrypsin levels, whereas other patients genetically deficient in α_1-antitrypsin are susceptible to hepatocellular carcinoma. No animal tumor models have been evaluated for the expression of α_1-antitrypsin.

The only species in which α_1-antitrypsin has been evaluated is man, and the only body fluid studied has been serum. The usual method of assay is rocket immunoelectrophoresis or electrophoresis followed by immunodiffusion. Increased serum α_1-antitrypsin has been associated with metastasizing bronchial carcinoma (Gropp and Havemann, 1980) and with overt lung metastasis (Coombes et al., 1977). α_1-Antitrypsin has also been associated with hepatocellular carcinoma; it was found to be elevated in 32 of the 39 (88.9%) patients examined (Chio and Oon, 1979). When α_1-antitrypsin and α_1-acid glycoprotein were evaluated together, it was possible to distinguish hepatocellular carcinoma from the benign liver diseases, cirrhosis and hepatitis (Chio and Oon, 1979). The presence of α_1-antitrypsin on the surface of hepatomas has been demonstrated using immunohistochemical techniques (Reintoft and Hagerstrand, 1979). Interestingly, two patients who were partially deficient in α_1-antitrypsin were found to have hepatocellular carcinoma postmortem. The discrepancy between this latter report and the increased α_1-antitrypsin reported above (Chio and Oon, 1979) remains unresolved.

The usefulness of α_1-antitrypsin as a tumor marker needs to be fully evaluated both in animals and in man. Studies relating α_1-antitrypsin levels to type of tumor, tumor burden, stage of disease, benign disease controls, and general population control levels should be performed.

EDC1 GLYCOPROTEIN

This glycopeptide is secreted in the urine of cancer patients with advanced neoplastic disease (Rudman et al., 1976). It is a proteolytic fragment derived from plasma inter-alpha trypsin inhibitor (Chawla et al., 1977). EDC1, consequently, is useful only for following the therapeutic course of the disease. It is of little or no value currently as an early cancer marker in humans, and its presence in animal tumors is unreported. EDC1 glycoprotein is detected using a radioimmunoassay.

PREGNANCY-SPECIFIC β_1-GLYCOPROTEIN

Pregnancy-specific β_1-glycoprotein (SP_1) is not a very reliable tumor marker, as it is expressed to varying extents by normal human tissues. It is, however, elevated in several types of cancer and thus may be useful for following the course of therapy. It is often found elevated along with human chorionic gonadotropin (HCG) which may be a superior cancer diagnostic aid. A radioimmunoassay is available for SP_1.

CELL-SURFACE GLYCOPROTEINS

There is much evidence suggesting that neoplastic cell transformation results in the altered expression of cell-surface glycoprotein structures. However, these alterations have primarily been associated with investigative research, but not with clinical or animal model studies of cancer. Therefore, the prospects of developing cell-surface glycoproteins as cancer markers lie ahead of us.

PREGNANCY-ASSOCIATED α_2-GLYCOPROTEIN

Pregnancy-associated α_2-glycoprotein (α_2-PAG or α_2-PAM) was found to be elevated in two separate breast cancer studies. Anderson et al. (1979) found α_2-PAG elevated more than 75% in 10 of 11 stage I or II breast cancer patients; Stimson (1978) reported an 85% correlation between increased α_2-PAG levels and recurrent breast cancer. Other types of cancer, including gynecologic cancer (Bauer and Krause, 1980) and ovarian cancer (Wuhan Medical College, Department of Pathophysiology, 1978), showed a reduced incidence of α_2-PAG elevation (60-70% of cancer patients showed an increase). The overall false-positive rate in the latter study of ovarian cancer was only 2.3%, but the incidence of increased α_2-PAG in benign disease was not reported. The test usually employed is a rapid, inexpensive, and simple radioimmuno-assay. α_2-PAG may be a useful marker for the detection of breast cancer. Wider population studies should be under-taken to evaluate more fully the statistics of increased α_2-PAG in breast cancer as well as to understand the false-positive results in the general population.

β_2-GLYCOPROTEIN

Alsabti and Muneir (1979) reported that β_2-glycoprotein was significantly elevated in 18 breast cancer patients pre-operatively, and that its levels correlated with the disease state three months postoperatively. β_2-Glycoprotein can be measured by radioimmunoassay and may be useful in the diagnosis and prognosis of breast cancer, but larger popula-tion studies are urged, particularly as a part of a multi-parameter cancer marker assessment. No animal studies have been reported.

SIALYL AND FUCOSYL GLYCOPEPTIDES

There is much evidence that sialyl and fucosyl glycopep-tides are altered in both animal and human tumors. However, these alterations are generally associated with cell-surface changes, necessitating tumor biopsies to establish the pres-ence of the alterations. (See the sections on glycosidases and blood carbohydrates and glycosyltransferases for a more complete discussion of fucose and sialic acid alterations associated with cancer.)

GLYCOLIPIDS

Numerous studies have demonstrated changes in glycolipid structure with transformation of cells to a neoplastic state. A loss of complex gangliosides and large glyco-lipids and the appearance of simpler gangliosides and glycolipids bearing shorter carbohydrate chains (reviewed by Yogeeswaran, 1980) have been observed. The glycolipid and ganglioside changes are associated with the cell sur-face, thereby limiting the usefulness of these changes as tumor markers. Tissue biopsies are required to identify the glycolipids and gangliosides. Their concentrations in

serum of cancer-bearing animals or patients have not been
evaluated and would involve a slow, labor-intensive procedure by qualified personnel. Glycolipids are usually
characterized by thin-layer chromatography.

TROPHOBLAST-SPECIFIC β_1-GLYCOPROTEIN

Trophoblast-specific β_1-glycoprotein is an excellent marker
for trophoblastic tumors (Tatarinov, 1978), yielding a
0% false-positive rate (except for pregnant women) and a
reported false negative rate of 20%. When other tumors are
assayed, the true positives are 30% and less, suggesting
that trophoblast-specific β_1-glycoprotein is not suitable
as a general cancer marker. The assay is a rapid, inexpensive radioimmunoassay that can be performed in most clinical
laboratories.

MAKARI'S TUMOR POLYSACCHARIDE ANTIGEN

Makari's tumor polysaccharide antigen is a potentially
useful marker. It was reported that 18% of reproductive
organ cancers were positive for this marker (Fishman et al.,
1975). The incidence of response to this antigen has not
been studied in the general population. The test is based
on a skin reaction that may be too complex to serve as a
marker.

TENNESSEE ANTIGEN

Tennessee antigen could be a useful tumor marker when used
in conjunction with other markers. Unfortunately, the assay
suffers from having a high false-positive rate in a healthy
general population (18%) and in other active lung and gastrointestinal disorders (29.5%) (Potter et al., 1980). The
assay sensitivity needs to be improved, the minimum tumor
burden for detection needs to be evaluated, and the cancer
specificity needs to be determined.

BJORKLUND'S TISSUE POLYPEPTIDE ANTIGEN

Bjorklund's tissue polypeptide antigen (TPA) is reported to
be a general marker for metastatic tumors; it is present in
73% of all cancer patients bearing metastatic tumors. TPA
was found in 54% of untreated primary tumor-bearing patients

and in 50% of ovarian tumor-bearing patients (Fishman et al., 1975). TPA is quantitated using a radioimmunoassay. No animal studies on the association of TPA and cancer have been reported.

HNC1β

HNC1β is a glycoprotein (MW 33,000) excreted into the urine of patients with disseminated cancer. An unidentified, antigenetically related, high-molecular-weight glycoprotein (MW 150,000) is present in approximately the same concentration in the plasma of normal and cancer patients (Rudman et al., 1978). HNC1β may also be related to EDC1 (Rudman et al., 1978). The elevated HNC1β levels in the urine of patients bearing disseminated cancer and having normal levels in the circulation leaves its urinary source unexplained. A radioimmunoassay is available for quantitating HNC1β. It would be advisable to examine this marker more thoroughly to establish its identity and origins. No animal studies that used HNC1β as a tumor marker have been reported.

Ca ANTIGEN

The Ca antigen, unique to human malignant tumors, was recently reported by Ashall et al. (1982). It appears to be a membrane-bound glycoprotein composed of two polypeptide chains with molecular weights of 390,000 and 350,000 daltons. Monoclonal antibodies directed toward the Ca antigen have been prepared and are used in a radioimmunoassay. Antibody binding could be inhibited by prior treatment of Ca antigen with neuraminidase, mixed endo- and exoglycosidases, keratin sulfate endo-β-galactosidase, and prolonged pronase digestion (the pronase used may contain unknown glycosidase activity). These results suggest that the specificity of Ca antigen may reside in the saccharide portion of the molecule but that the protein may also be important for specificity.

McGee et al. (1982) examined various normal, benign, and malignant human tissue sections immunohistochemically. The majority of the malignant tumors expressed the Ca antigen, but several significant exceptions were noted, including prostatic carcinomas, testicular teratocarcinomas and seminomas, some sarcomas, some lymphomas, malignant brain tumors, neuroblastomas, and melanomas. Ca antigen was least readily detected in epithelial malignancies of the alimentary tract, particularly of the colon. Normal tissues in which Ca antigen was detected were the epithelium of the fallopian tube and transitional epithelium of the urinary tract. Ca antigen was not detected on any benign tumors. Although the Ca antigen was found in tumor effusates, no studies of Ca antigen in urine, blood, or cerebrospinal fluid were reported.

This relatively new marker for human malignant tumors needs further substantiation. Studies require wider population testing to ascertain its association with specific tumor types, its time of appearance, its presence in readily accessible body fluids, and evaluation of false-positive and false-negative results.

The Ca antigen was reported to be present in the mouse cell line PG19, from a spontaneous melanoma of a C57 black mouse (Ashall et al., 1982). No other reports of the Ca antigen in animals were noted.

GLYCOPROTEINS DETERMINED TO BE CURRENTLY UNPROVEN AS MARKERS

Table X-1 shows the glycoproteins that were deemed to have insufficient support at this time for further consideration as cancer markers in animal screens and indicates the reason why each is so evaluated.

Table X-1

GLYCOPROTEINS DETERMINED TO REQUIRE
FURTHER STUDY AS POTENTIAL CANCER MARKERS

Compound	Comment	References
TSH	Elevated in only 30% of patients, high false negatives	Dunzendorfer et al., 1981
Blood group antigen	Has not been evaluated for association or prevalence of alteration with cancer; still in research stage	Yogeeswaran, 1980; Watanabe and Hakomori, 1976
Galactosyltransferase acceptor	Inhibits growth of tumor cells in culture, but no association with tumor cells developed	Podolsky and Isselbacher, 1980
JBB5	High false negatives (67%)	Chawla et al., 1977
Tumor-specific soluble mammary tumor glycoprotein	Not found in sera of breast cancer patients	Leung and Edgington, 1980
α-Mouse mammary tumor glycoprotein	Mouse virus antigen found in human tumor	Ohno et al., 1979

XI

Hormones as Tumor Markers

A. Winship-Ball, C.T. Helmes, J.P. Miller, H.L. Johnson

INTRODUCTION

Hormones are particularly attractive as potential markers of
preneoplastic and neoplastic events in man because they are
easily sampled in blood, urine, or tissue biopsies, and can
be analyzed relatively inexpensively by radioimmunoassay or
enzyme-bridge immunoperoxidase techniques. However, equivalent studies in animals have not been pursued extensively.
Almost all biologically active protein and polypeptide hormones have been eutopically or ectopically produced in a
wide variety of neoplastic conditions in men and women
(Fenoglio, 1980). In endocrine tumors, the hormone produced
is generally immunologically identical with the physiologic
hormone, and clinical syndromes may develop. In nonendo-
crine tumors, the hormones or hormone fragments produced
may be immunologically similar to physiologic hormones also,
but they are often nonfunctional, and secondary clinical
syndromes are unusual (Lokich, 1978). An exception is "Big"
ACTH, which is metabolized to a biologically active form.
Table XI-1 summarizes information available on the eutopic
and ectopic production of a variety of hormonal secretions
in humans, some of which are discussed in greater detail.

Although the actual mechanism of ectopic hormone production
is unknown, the most popular theories concern production
by

- Amine precursor uptake and decarboxylation (APUD)
  cells distributed throughout the body.

110

Table XI-1

HORMONES ASSOCIATED WITH TUMORS IN HUMANS

Hormone	Tumor Association	References
Parathyrin	Parathyroid adenomas and carcinomas; tumors of the kidney, lung, liver, adrenals, parotids; renal adenocarcinomas; breast carcinoma; epidermoid carcinoma of the lung; squamous cell tumors; oat cell carcinoma of the lung	Bagshawe and Searle (1977) Griffing and Vaitukaitis (1980)
Calcitonin	Medullary thyroid cancer, cancer of the pancreas; tumors of the prostate, breast; pheochromocytoma, oat cell cancer of the lung; tumors of pancreas and uterus, parathyroid hyperplasia and adenoma, carcinoid	Silva and Becker (1978) Bagshawe and Searle (1977) Sizemore et al. (1977) Milhaud et al. (1977) Gropp et al. (1980) Neville et al. (1976) Coombes et al. (1977) Coombes (1980) Waalkes and Tormey (1978)
Insulin	Insulinoma, various lymphosarcomas and other sarcomas, bronchogenic tumors, fibrosarcomas, retroperitoneal tumors, leiomyosarcomas,	Bagshawe and Searle (1977) Lokich (1978) Rees (1975)

(Continued)

Table XI-1 (Continued)

Hormone	Tumor Association	References
	hemangiopericytomas, carcinoma of the cervix	Bagshawe and Searle (1977)
Catecholamines	Pheochromocytoma; tumors of the spleen, breast, and testis	Covington et al. (1974)
Vanillylmandelic acid	Neuroblastoma, pheochromocytoma, ganglioneuroma, ganglioblastoma	
Vasopressin (antidiuretic hormone)	Oat cell carcinoma of the lung, Ewing's sarcoma, adenocarcinoma of the pancreas, bronchial carcinoid, papillary carcinoma of the duodenum	Bagshawe and Searle (1977) Ishikawa et al. (1980) Coombes et al. (1978)
Neurophysin	Oat cell carcinoma of the lung	Griffing and Vaitukaitis (1980) Rees (1975) Ishikawa et al. (1980)
Oxytocin	Oat cell carcinoma of the lung	Ishikawa et al. (1980) Griffing and Vaitukaitis (1980) Rees (1975)

(Continued)

Table XI-1 (Continued)

Hormone	Tumor Association	References
Prolactin	Tumors of the endometrium, kidney, lung, ovary, prostate, pituitary, breast (human and rat), testis (human and rat); urogenital cancer	Hagen et al. (1979)
Growth hormone	Tumors of the pituitary, lung, ovary, stomach, breast (human and canine)	Hagen et al. (1979)
Thyrotropin (thyroid stimulating hormone)	Pituitary tumors, urogenital cancer	Hagen et al. (1979) Bagshawe and Searle (1977)
Adrenocortico-tropin	Pituitary adenoma and carcinoma, oat cell carcinoma of the lung, carcinoid, thymoma, pheochromocytoma, tumors of the colon, pancreas, medullary thyroid, prostate, cervix, ovary; neuroblastoma	Griffing and Vaitukaitis (1980) Bagshawe and Searle (1977) Rees (1975) Ishikawa et al. (1980) Homma (1980) Gropp and Havemann (1980)

(Continued)

Table XI-1 (Continued)

Hormone	Tumor Association	References
Follicle-stimulating hormone	Pituitary adenoma; adenocarcinoma of the prostate and interstitial cell tumors of the testis (rats); ovarian tumors (mice)	Griffing and Vaitukaitis (1980) Snyder et al. (1980) Takeuchi et al. (1980) Brown et al. (1979)
Luteinizing hormone	Adenocarcinoma of prostate and interstitial cell tumors of the testis (rats); ovarian tumors (mice)	Brown et al. (1979) Ylikorkala et al. (1979) Foss et al. (1980)
Placental protein five	Hydatidiform mole; cancer of the breast, genitourinary tract, gastrointestinal tract	Inaba et al. (1980) Samaan et al. (1976) Horne and Bremner (1980) Seppala et al. (1979)
Placental protein ten	Tumors of the breast, testis, ovaries, endometrium, gastrointestinal tract	Inaba et al. (1980) Horne and Bremner (1980)
Placental protein eleven	Tumors of the heart, testis, ovarian endometrium, gastrointestinal tract	Inaba et al. (1980)
Placental protein twelve	Tumors of the heart, testis, ovarian endometrium, gastrointestinal tract	Inaba et al. (1980)

(Continued)

Table XI-1 (Continued)

Hormone	Tumor Association	References
Placental anemia inducing factor	Nonspecific	Oh-Uti et al. (1980)
SP_1	Trophoblastic tumors; nontrophoblastic tumors of the lung, breast, gastrointestinal tract	Inaba et al. (1980) Lee et al. (1981)
SP_3 (pregnancy-associated glycoprotein)	Malignant melanoma; cancer of the breast, lung, colon	Bagshawe and Searle (1977)
Chorionic thyrotropin	Nonspecific	Anderson (1979) Rees (1975)
Chorionic gonadotropin	Hydatidiform and invasive mole; gestational choriocarcinoma; malignant teratoma; hepatocellular carcinoma; tumors of the lung, breast, gastrointestinal tract	Bagshawe and Searle (1977) Tormey et al., (1979) Farrell (1980) Rochman (1979) Fishman et al. (1975) Kirschner et al., (1981) Anderson (1979) Kamidona et al. (1980)

(Continued)

Table XI-1 (Concluded)

Hormone	Tumor Association	References
Human placental lactogen	Hydatidiform and invasive mole; gestational choriocarcinoma, malignant teratoma, hepatocellular carcinoma, germ-cell tumors of the testis, bronchogenic carcinoma, ovarian carcinoma, breast cancer, cancer of the prostate	Javadpour (1979) Lee et al. (1981) Bagshawe and Searle (1977) Rosen et al. (1975) Szymandera et al. (1981) Broder et al. (1977) Horne et al. (1976) Rees (1975) Samaan et al. (1976) Stanhope et al. (1979) Coombes et al. (1978) Homma (1980)
Vasoactive intestinal peptide	Pancreatic islet cell tumors	Bloom et al. (1973)

- Transformed differentiated somatic cells whose functions have been altered as a result of derepression of early expressed genes.

- Cell lines from transformed pluripotential progenitors, differing in degree of differentiation and thus in hormones and antigens produced (Baylin and Mendelsohn, 1980). This theory of "dysdifferentiation" accounts for the development of both monoclonal and differentiated tumors and provides a basis for the ectopic production of any hormone.

The hormones most commonly produced ectopically are the peptides--ACTH, calcitonin, ADH, PTH, HCG, and prolactin. The synthesis of ectopic glycoproteins (e.g., LH, TSH, FSH) is less frequent--except in the case of pregnancy-associated proteins. Ectopic production of steroids and thyroid hormones is rare, presumably because of the complexity of synthesis.

The presence or absence of hormone receptors--particularly estrogen and progesterone receptors in breast tumors--has also been used as an indicator of neoplasia and as a tool in evaluating prognosis and determining therapeutic strategies. Although it was once believed that only malignant tissue contained significant numbers of estrogen and progesterone receptors, it is now commonly accepted that both apparently healthy and transformed tissues in various parts of the body may contain receptors; the particular significance of the quantity and distribution of steroid receptors has not been established.

However, the purpose of this review was to determine the potential utility of various hormones as markers of carcinogenesis in animal screens.

The overwhelming majority of papers reviewed consisted of analyses of human serum or tumor cytosol for differentiating tumor types, for clinical staging, or for detecting tumor recurrence or metastasis. A small number of papers concerned the presence or absence of hormone receptors in humans; an even smaller number reported the results of experimental animal studies. The criteria used in evaluating the potential utility of a marker include

- The specificity, sensitivity, and accuracy of the marker.

- The temporal relationship between detection of the marker and diagnosis of a preneoplastic or early neoplastic condition.

- The relationship, if any, between hormonal markers in humans and laboratory animals.

The attempt to identify tumor markers of potential use in bioassays was made very difficult by the fact that virtually no data on hormonal markers of carcinogenesis in animals are available. Data on humans have been collected principally from various hospitalized populations, and true baseline or control values may not have been determined. Most such studies have been retrospective; the malignant condition was diagnosed before the marker was detected. Few patients have been identified in "preneoplastic" or early stages of neoplastic disease. Therefore, although many of the markers identified by clinical monitoring are useful in surveillance and detection of more advanced stages of disease, their diagnostic value in early stages appears to be limited.

HORMONAL MARKERS OF INTEREST IN ANIMAL STUDIES

The detection of hormonal tumor markers in experimental animals appears to have been largely ignored. Fewer than ten such studies were reported; none concerned hormones currently used in the diagnosis or therapeutic management of human cancer patients. The animal studies that are of possible interest concern diethylstilbestrol (DES), progesterone, follicle-stimulating hormone (FSH), and luteinizing hormone (LH).

Progesterone

A study by Aussel et al. (1979) is of interest because a drop in progesterone levels was observed long before tumors developed. Pathogen-free female Sprague-Dawley female rats (N = 70) were administered N-2-fluorenylacetamide (FAA), a potent liver carcinogen, in a protein- and riboflavin-deficient synthetic diet. Synthetic-diet controls (N = 70) and controls fed an adequate diet (N = 70) were also maintained. Four rats from each group were serially sacrificed at intervals over a 200-day period, and serum samples were analyzed by radioimmunoassay for progesterone and estradiol levels. After two days of treatment, the penetration of hepatic cells by FAA was detected by fluorescence microscopy;

simultaneously, alpha-fetoprotein (AFP) was detected in the serum. After 20 days of treatment, FAA-treated rats exhibited a sharp drop in progesterone levels, while estradiol levels remained normal (Stora et al., 1981). The drop in progesterone levels, which predated the appearance of liver tumors by 130 days (Milano et al., 1981), was attributed to the production of AFP. The authors suggest that binding to estradiol inhibited estrogen catabolism, causing cessation of estrus and a concomitant drop in corpora lutea and progesterone production. To ensure that the observed fall in progesterone levels was due to AFP-estradiol binding, and not to toxicity to the ovaries, the investigators injected rats with AFP (Aussel et al., 1981). The results of this study were not available at the time this review was written; however, even if progesterone levels are due to increased AFP production, it is not obvious that an advantage would be derived from monitoring progesterone rather than AFP.

Follicle-Stimulating Hormone and Luteinizing Hormone

Follicle-stimulating hormone (FSH) and luteinizing hormone (LH), glycoproteins produced by the anterior pituitary under the direction of the hypothalamus, regulate the development, reproductive functions, and hormonal secretions of the ovary and testis. Eutopic FSH secretion has been associated with pituitary adenoma in vivo (Snyder et al., 1980) and in vitro (Takeuchi et al., 1980); ectopic production is rare. No consistent relationship between FSH or LH values and endometrial, ovarian (Ylikorkala et al., 1979), or testicular germ cell tumors (Foss et al., 1980) in humans was reported in the literature reviewed, but two experimental animal studies are of interest. In the first, normal intact male pathogen-free NEDH rats were parabiosed to castrated males or oophorectomized females. The appearance of interstitial cell tumors of the testis and adenocarcinomas of the prostate in intact male rats was preceded by elevations of FSH and LH in the sera of castrated males or oophorectomized females and high levels of testosterone and androstenedione in the target members developing tumors (Brown et al., 1979). In the second study, high FSH, LH, and PRL levels preceded the development of ovarian tumors in thymectomized mice (Michael et al., 1981). By the time tumors appeared, however, the FSH and LH levels were low.

In both studies, high FSH and LH levels were predictive of tumor development. Although the assays require more manipulation than may be desirable in an ideal short-term animal test, the inclusion of LH and FSH in biochemical screens for carcinogenicity in animal assays might be of some value.

HORMONAL MARKERS OF INTEREST IN HUMAN STUDIES

The three hormones most useful in the diagnosis of human cancer are calcitonin, chorionic gonadotrophin, and desmosterol. None has been systematically investigated in animals.

Calcitonin

Calcitonin, a normal product of C-cells of the thyroid gland, regulates concentrations of calcium in the circulating blood. It is secreted eutopically in medullary thyroid carcinoma (Milhaud et al., 1977; Neville et al., 1976), Cushing's syndrome, pheochromocytoma, and parathyroid hyperplasia and adenoma (Bagshawe and Searle, 1977). It is secreted ectopically in bronchogenic carcinoma--particularly oat cell carcinoma (Gropp and Havemann, 1980)--breast cancer (Coombes, 1980; Coombes et al., 1977; Waalkes et al., 1978), and various tumors of the pancreas, prostate, and uterus (Bagshawe and Searle, 1977).

No data from animal tests were available; therefore, calcitonin's usefulness in bioassays cannot be predicted. However, calcitonin appears to be an excellent marker in medullary thyroid carcinoma (MTC). Calcitonin levels are increased in approximately 75% of patients with MTC, even when no palpable mass is present (Bagshawe and Searle, 1977). In a five-year prospective study of a population at risk of medullary thyroid carcinoma (MTC), 90% of 72 individuals with MTC or C-cell hyperplasia were detected by radioimmunoassay using plasma immunoreactive calcitonin (Sizemore et al., 1977). The presence of histaminase indicated a neoplastic rather than a hyperplastic condition. Elevated serum calcitonin levels are also common in metastatic breast cancer, oat cell cancer of the lung, and carcinoid tumors (Rees, 1975). Although some investigators disagree (Silva and Becker, 1978; Rosen, 1981), the consensus appears to be that elevated serum calcitonin (greater than 3000 pg/ml) is a useful marker for the early detection of familial and nonfamilial MTC (Sizemore et al., 1977); the simultaneous detection of histaminase may indicate the presence of more malignant forms of the disease (Baylin and Mendelsohn, 1980). Heterogeneous forms of calcitonin and variable site specificity of antisera have led to substantial variation in radioimmunoassay results from different laboratories. Therefore, determination of the usefulness of calcitonin as a marker in animal tests for carcinogenesis may depend in part on the development of reliable assay techniques.

Human Chorionic Gonadotropin (HCG)

Human chorionic gonadotropin (HCG) is a glycoprotein trophic hormone similar in structure to luteinizing hormone (LH), follicle-stimulating hormone (FSH), and thyroid-stimulating hormone (TSH). All have a common quaternary structure of two dissimilar, noncovalently linked subunits. The four hormones have virtually identical alpha subunits (Griffing and Vaitukaitis, 1980); the beta subunit of each hormone is unique and is responsible for the hormone's specificity. Clinical assays performed by many investigators cannot distinguish between HCG and LH because of their structural similarity. In contrast, radioimmunoassays using an antibody to the beta subunit of HCG can selectively detect HCG in the presence of LH or other glycoprotein trophic hormones (Vaitukaitis et al., 1972). Beta-HCG is an excellent marker of trophoblastic tumors in males. It is easily detected in the urine before the appearance of clinical signs of cancer. As a marker of testicular choriocarcinoma, it has a sensitivity of 100%; it can indicate tumor masses of 10^4 to 10^6 cells (Farrell, 1980). As a marker of testicular germ-cell tumors, HCG has a false-positive rate of 0% (Rosen et al., 1975; Javadpour, 1979; Kamidono et al., 1980). HCG is considerably less useful as a cancer marker in women because it is associated with pregnancy, hydatidiform mole, and other gynecologic conditions, including benign ovarian and breast tumors. Its sensitivity as a marker of ovarian and cervical cancer is low--approximately 43% and 60%, respectively (Fishman et al., 1975; Bhattacharya and Barlow, 1979; Samaan et al., 1976; Farrell, 1980).

HCG is a poor marker of nontrophoblastic tumors (Rochman, 1978; Kirschner et al., 1981) and would not be an accurate predictor of cancer in the general population (Braunstein, 1981). Nevertheless, it is useful in the detection of trophoblastic tumors in males. In the absence of experimental evidence, its utility as a tumor marker in laboratory animals cannot be evaluated, but it is worthy of investigation.

The inclusion of chorionic gonadotropin in a multiparametric screen might be a useful addition to protocols for carcinogenesis bioassays.

Desmosterol

Desmosterol, the immediate precursor of cholesterol in the pathway of brain sterol synthesis, is not normally detected in the cerebrospinal fluid (CSF) of mature individuals; it is elevated in the CSF of a high percentage of patients with primary but not metastatic brain tumors (Wasserstrom et al., 1981). The test for desmosterol requires an oral dose of 500 mg of triparanol for five days, followed by lumbar puncture. The conditions of the test and the low prevalence of brain tumors in the general population (0.005%) preclude its use as a routine screen (Seidenfeld and Marton, 1978,1979). However, in a population with neurologic symptoms and an assumed prevalence of 25%, its predictive value is estimated to be 95%.

CONCLUSIONS AND RECOMMENDATIONS FOR RESEARCH

Except in isolated instances (calcitonin in MTC and HCG in trophoblastic tumors), the identification and measurement of endocrine markers in humans has not facilitated the early diagnosis of malignancy (Baylin and Mendelsohn, 1980), although hormones have proved to be useful in clinical staging, tumor differentiation, and monitoring of cancer patients. The significance of hormonal markers of carcinogenesis in laboratory animals has scarcely been addressed. Markers that predict, rather than merely reflect, carcinogenesis are of particular interest, as are markers that enable detection of tumors in early stages of development. Chorionic gonadotropin, calcitonin, progesterone, FSH, and LH are potentially useful markers that might be monitored in carcinogenesis bioassays.

The addition of serial multiparametric screens for hormonal and nonhormonal markers to protocols for animal studies of carcinogenesis might permit early detection of tumors and characterization of products of transformed cells over the course of disease. Serial screens in species with high spontaneous tumor incidence might provide information on markers associated with the development of spontaneous tumors; by exposing the same species to chemical carcinogens one could detect similarities and differences in biochemical markers or the number and distribution of hormone receptors in both "spontaneous" and chemically induced carcinogenesis.

Although DES is not itself a marker, the use of this animal model of transplacental carcinogenesis--specifically the monitoring of progeny for markers of subsequent carcinogenesis--might be worthy of some effort. Chronic treatment with diethylstilbestrol (DES) results in low to high incidence of pituitary tumors in rats, depending on the strain. Chronic intrauterine exposure to DES is associated with genital abnormalities in animal species (female monkeys and mice) and with the development of clear-cell adenocarcinoma of the vagina and cervix in female human progeny.

XII

Immunological and Oncodevelopmental Markers

R.M. Miao, M.J. Lipsett, L.T. Juhos, W.E. Davis, P.Y. Fung

INTRODUCTION

Immunologic markers are changes in the components of the immune system that are associated with premalignancy, malignancy, or tumor recurrence. Immunologic markers do not include systems that use immunologic techniques (e.g., antigen-antibody reactions, complement-fixation) to detect antigens that have been characterized biochemically, such as enzymes and cell surface proteins or glycoproteins.

It is the purpose of this review to identify and evaluate those immunologic markers that have been or might be diagnostic of tumor progression (tumor development) as opposed to those that have been used for the identification of already-developed tumors.

There have been few studies reported on the detection of immunologic markers in man or in experimental animals. Most such reports have been of clinical studies concerned with the identification of immune components in leukemias and lymphomas or in the immunologic detection of tumor-associated antigens of unknown function. Such studies have not been concerned with the identification of immunologic markers and will, therefore, be described here only briefly. In addition, the extensive literature on carcinoembryonic antigen (CEA) will be dealt with summarily. The considerable literature dealing with leukemic and solid tumor-associated antigens and with viral antigens associated with some forms of cancer cannot be critically evaluated because little, if any, data are available on their relationship to

early stages of tumor progression in humans. The identification of tumor-associated antigens (leukemic and solid
tumors) has been used principally to identify the specific
cell types involved in various forms of cancer. These antigens should obviously be studied to determine whether any of
them are associated with tumor progression. The paucity of
data on correlations between tumor-associated antigens and
tumor progression, however, places this area of research at
its inception. To recommend specific research projects in
this area would require development of proposals based upon
scant or nonexistent data. This is obviously fertile ground
for future investigations. Readers are referred to two
excellent works dealing with immunodiagnosis of cancers for
evaluation of presently known tumor cell antigens (Herberman
and McIntire, 1979; Ungerleider, 1981).

At least three immunologic markers of tumorigenesis warrant
further investigation at this time: α-fetoprotein (AFP),
leukocyte adherence inhibition, and circulating immune
complexes.

α-FETOPROTEIN (AFP)

The α-globulin, α-fetoprotein, is normally present in
high concentration in fetal blood and in low concentration
in adult blood. Elevations in adult blood appear to be
related to yolk-sac (endodermal sinus) teratocarcinomas
of the gonads or to hepatocellular carcinomas. Therefore,
increased concentrations of circulating AFP in adult blood
may be significant in the diagnosis of cancer at those
sites. Also, changes in the concentrations of circulating
AFP assist in evaluating the prognosis and therapeutic
response in the clinical management of these tumors (Adinolfi, 1979; Sell and Becker, 1978). Whereas no documented
examples were found in the literature of exposures of humans
to known chemical hepatocarcinogens that included measured
increases in circulating AFP, there are several such examples in rodent species following exposure to a variety of
chemical agents.

AFP could serve as a cancer marker if more were known about
the details of chronology of carcinogenicity after exposure
to known carcinogens.

Animal Studies

The use of AFP as a marker of neoplastic activity in

animals includes its identification (Abelev, 1963), isolation (Sell, 1972), characterization of its structure (Watabe, 1974), binding capacity (Ruoslahti, 1978; Soloff, 1971), and immunological properties (Ruoslahti, 1975). The age-dependent, normal values of circulating AFP and their alterations resulting from a variety of liver injuries (partial hepatectomy, administration of toxic and carcinogenic agents, hepatoma transplantation and its subsequent surgical manipulations) were shown to occur in the rat (Sell, 1978). Insight was gained into some aspects of the molecular biology concerning the relation of mRNA, the associated translation process, and the circulating levels of AFP with transplanted hepatomas in rats (Sell, 1974,1977,1978; Sala-Trepat, 1979; Wepsic, 1978). Immunological treatment using anti-AFP preparations reduced the growth of transplanted hepatomas (Mizejewski, 1974) and of hepatomas produced by exposure of rats to 4-dimethylaminoazobenzene (DAB) (Hirai, 1982). The use of improved analytic techniques in several studies allowed the kinetic patterns of AFP production to be described in rats as they responded to selected hepatocarcinogens (Sell, 1979,1982). Four different patterns of hepatocellular response were shown when induced by either diethylnitrosamine (DEN), DAB, N-2-fluorenylacetamide (FAA) or ethionine and azaserine. In these model systems, neoplastic nodules and hepatomas were produced experimentally with circulating levels of AFP increasing to various extents for variable durations and different times according to the carcinogen administered. Diets deficient in lipotropes, fed during carcinogen exposure, repeatedly increased circulating AFP levels in rats repeatedly (Leffert, 1977; Shinozuka, 1979). The pattern of AFP response in mice during neoplastic development differs from that found in rats, in that the early appearance of AFP is not shown by mice fed hepatocarcinogens.

Animal studies, principally in rats, show that several agents produce liver injury or hepatocarcinomas that result in elevated levels of circulating AFP. Among these are galactosamine (Sell et al., 1976), phenobarbital (Smuckler et al., 1975), ethionine (Hancock et al., 1975), 4-dimethylaminobenzene (Watabe et al., 1973), FAA (Kitigawa et al., 1972), azo dyes (Onoe et al., 1973), DEN (Watabe, 1971), and benzo(α)pyrene (Boyd et al., 1981). The experience with benzo(α)pyrene (Boyd et al., 1981) and the use of additional testing for mutagens in urine (Salmonella/mammalian microsome test) show that multiple indicators can be used for the early detection of carcinogenesis.

In most studies, AFP assays were performed with goat antiserum specific against rat AFP. A persistent problem
demanding clarification is the species-specificity of the
antisera used in animal studies; their relevance to human
studies is even more obscure. From experiments with transplantable rat hepatomas, the AFP concentration in the serum
and the AFP content in the hepatoma cells were correlated,
presumably because both sources reflect synthesis of AFP
by the hepatomas (Sell et al., 1979) and/or "oval" cells
(Sell and Leffert, 1982). Cellular AFP production is considered to be caused by altered regulation of gene expression of fetal proteins in stem cells. The correlation
between the rapid growth rate of a tumor or the degree of
abnormal chromosome composition and the corresponding rate
of AFP production remains to be defined. Future research
with animals could clarify these points.

Human Studies

In clinical practice, AFP measurements are used as diagnostic criteria, in prognosis, or in monitoring the therapy of
already diagnosed cancer. In no instance of human cancer
has the increment in circulating AFP been associated with
a documented history of exposure to a known carcinogen.
Certainly there are conditions, not immediately associated
with carcinogenicity, of the presence of increased circulating levels of AFP (pregnancy, hepatitis, cirrhosis
of the liver). The normal concentration of AFP in adult
human serum is less than 5 ng/ml. Concentrations greater
than 1000 ng/ml are diagnostic of an AFP-producing tumor.
Values between 5 and 1000 ng/ml require additional diagnostic techniques to establish or refute neoplastic activity.
Sustained, increased levels of circulating AFP strongly
suggest a tumor burden (Sell, 1980). The wide range of
uncertainty (5 to 1000 ng/ml) between normalcy and definite
evidence of neoplastic activity renders AFP questionable
as an early marker of carcinogenesis, but defines the
concentration range of AFP on which future research must
dwell. Modern technologies (such as the use of monoclonal
antibodies) may be attractive ways with which to explore
this gray area and with which to increase the specificity
and sensitivity of future diagnostic techniques for measuring AFP.

LEUKOCYTE ADHERENCE INHIBITION

The leukocyte adherence inhibition (LAI) assay was first

described by Halliday and Miller (1972). It is based on the observation that, when sensitized leukocytes react with the corresponding antigen, their normal adherence to glass is inhibited. Not all leukocytes adhere to glass. Goldrosen et al. (1979) reported that sensitized monocytes are the responsive cells in LAI assays and that neither T- nor B-lymphocytes respond in LAI tests. Recently, however, Bekesi et al. (1982) reported that T-lymphocytes are responsive in the LAI assay, at least for breast tumors. Furthermore, they reported that removing B-lymphocytes and monocytes from test sera eliminated nonspecific LAI responses to several unrelated tumor antigens. These results need to be confirmed, because T-lymphocytes do not normally adhere to glass. At the present time, it appears that monocytes and, in certain situations, T-lymphocytes respond in the LAI test.

The micro-LAI assay appears to be the most suitable for reproducibility, standardization, and large-scale applications. In this assay, antigens and leukocytes are added to individual wells in 24-well microtest plates. After an hour of incubation, nonadherent leukocytes are gently removed by washing, and adherent leukocytes are fixed, stained, and counted using an automated differential scanning system. The usual antigens in this assay are crude cell membrane preparations from tumors, normal tissues, and nontumorous diseased tissue. Either peritoneal or circulating leukocytes may be employed. Monocytes preserved by freezing in liquid nitrogen, with DMSO as a cryopreservative, appear to be as sensitive as freshly prepared monocytes in the LAI assay (Waldman and Yonemoto, 1978). Freeze-storage does not appear to affect either the monocytes' specificity or sensitivity to various antigens. The ability to store monocytes is important for long-term studies such as in vivo carcinogenicity tests in animals; rather than comparing data obtained at different times using different antigen preparations, it is possible to compare several monocyte preparations from the same animal or patient at one time against the same antigen preparation.

The source of specific antigen need not be the same as the source of sensitized leukocytes. The monocyte-antigen reaction is tissue-specific. Leukocytes from patients with pancreatic carcinomas will react with crude membrane preparations from pancreatic tumors from different donors but will not react with preparations from colon tumors or normal pancreas (Russo et al., 1978; Goldrosen et al., 1979;

Tataryn et al., 1978). Tumor-specific reactions also occur in animals bearing transplantable tumors. Leukocytes from mice (C57BL/6J) bearing transplantable B16 melanoma cells will react with B16 cell membranes but not with MCA-38 colon adenocarcinoma cell membranes (Leveson et al., 1977). Goldrosen et al. (1979) have shown that in C57BL/6J mice, MCA-38-sensitized B-cells (B-lymphocytes) can "program" normal monocytes to undergo MCA-38 antigen-induced adherence inhibition. In this situation, sensitized B-cells appear to excrete a soluble mediator, which may be an immunoglobulin. In mice, B-lymphocytes might be sensitized by tumor antigens and produce an immunoglobulin mediator that sensitizes monocytes. Sensitized monocytes are then able to bind tumor antigens and are inhibited from adhering to glass (Goldrosen et al., 1979). Sarlo and Mortensen (1982) recently showed that sensitized T-lymphocytes from tumor-bearing mice produce a factor that decreases the adherence of monocytes in the LAI test. The factor is produced by spleen T-lymphocytes in mice with regressing murine-sarcoma-virus induced tumors. Both Lyt-1 and Lyt-2 positive T-cells produce this factor. Whether this T-lymphocyte factor is the same as the B-lymphocyte immunoglobulin mediator remains to be determined. Different lymphocyte subsets might be responsive to different antigens and produce LAI factors that act on various monocyte subsets.

The strength of the LAI assay as an early marker of tumorigenesis lies in the specificity of the monocyte-tumor membrane reaction (Leveson et al., 1977; Goldrosen et al., 1981; Ayeni et al., 1980; Thomson, 1979) and in the detection of sensitized monocytes well in advance of palpable tumors as in mice after the transplantation of an extremely small number of tumor cells (Leveson et al., 1977). Of particular significance is the study of Leveson et al. (1977) in which inoculating 5×10^3 B16 melanoma cells into C57BL/6J mice yielded LAI detection of tumor-antigen-sensitized leukocytes ten days after inoculation and 16 days before a palpable tumor appeared. These results suggest that LAI may be a highly sensitive early detection method for tumorigenesis in animal models.

Clinical investigations have shown that the LAI assay can identify tumor-antigen-sensitized leukocytes in at least three types of cancers--pancreatic (Russo et al., 1978; Goldrosen et al., 1981; Tataryn et al., 1978), mammary (Ayeni et al., 1980; Waldman and Yonemoto, 1978; Fujisawa

et al., 1977; Armitstead and Gowland, 1975), and gastrointestinal (Waldman and Yonemoto, 1978; Ayeni et al., 1980;
Halliday et al., 1977; Armitstead and Gowland, 1975; Maluish, 1979). Overall statistics indicate that the level of
sensitivity for the LAI procedure is greater than 85% and
the level of false positives is less than 5%. For example,
in assays involving patients with pancreatic tumors, the
data from combined studies show that 69 of 78 patients were
positive (88%) while 19 of 622 controls were false positive
(3%). The control groups included healthy individuals and
patients with acute pancreatitis, nonpancreatic malignant
tumors, benign tumors, and inflammatory diseases of the
colorectum, stomach, or lung (Russo et al., 1978; Goldrosen
et al., 1979; Tataryn et al., 1978; Ayeni et al., 1980).

In a number of clinical studies, as well as in those with
transplantable tumors in mice, the LAI assay is less sensitive in cases of greatest tumor progression. Leukocytes
from patients with advanced disease or metastases are less
sensitive to specific tumor antigens (Tataryn et al., 1978;
Goldrosen et al., 1981). The degree of false-positive
responses is still low, but the sensitivity of the assay
drops significantly (>85% vs <60%). In mice bearing B16
melanoma cells, the LAI assay fails to show any significant
leukocyte sensitivity when the tumor diameter reaches 1.5 cm
(Leveson et al., 1977). The reason for this is unclear. It
is possible that tumor antigens become masked or deleted or
that blocking antibodies are elicited that cannot sensitize
monocytes. This phenomenon may be related to the observation that sera from some patients and animals with progressive tumors contain a soluble blocking factor. The blocking
factor abrogates the reaction between sensitized leukocytes
and the specific tumor-membrane extracts. Not all patients
have blocking factors, and the relationship of blocking
factors to tumorigenesis is still unclear.

There is a significant limitation to the LAI assay. Sensitized leukocytes show specificity for tumor types, e.g.,
pancreatic vs breast tumors. This means that specific tumor
extracts must be available for the assay. This limitation
may not be insurmountable, because the source of the tumor
apparently is unimportant--leukocytes from one patient react
with antigens from a similar tumor in another patient. It
would seem highly unlikely that all pancreatic cancers arose
from the same causative events or agents. Therefore, the
high degree of sensitivity and the large population of

patients studied suggest that the causative event(s) or
chemical(s) leading to tumorigenesis are unimportant for
the LAI assay. The LAI assay, therefore, may be able to
detect tumorigenesis caused by diverse agents. Its use as
an early detection procedure in tumorigenesis is limited
by the need to obtain membrane antigens from tumors of
different tissues.

Several areas should be studied to validate the LAI assay
in animal models of tumorigenesis. While the results
reported by Leveson et al. (1977) show that the LAI assay
can detect very small tumor burdens, it must still be determined whether the assay can be used to detect chemically
induced tumors before palpable tumors appear. Studies
should be conducted on the role of immunoglobulin mediators
and T-lymphocyte factors in sensitizing monocytes to tumor
antigens. Characterization of mediators and elucidation of
the role of T- and B-lymphocytes during tumorigenesis may
be important for developing protocols and for immunotherapy
and for detecting sensitized monocytes. It would also help
in determining the mechanism causing decreased monocyte
reactivity as the tumor burden increases.

The overall evidence shows that the LAI assay can be used
to detect the early occurrence of tumors. The sensitivity
and specificity of the procedure are favorable. The ability
to perform large numbers of replicate assays and the low
cost and speed warrant further investigation of the LAI
assay as one part of a battery of tests for tumorigenesis.

IMMUNE COMPLEXES

Humoral factors, thought to consist of circulating immune
complexes (ICs), have been reported to block antitumor cell-
mediated cytotoxicity in vitro (Sjögren et al., 1971, 1972;
Baldwin and Robins, 1976). Such ICs have been detected
in cancer patients, as well as in noncancer patients with
autoimmune disease. (Theofilopoulous, 1977; Lancet, 1977;
Filliland and Mannik, 1977). At least 18 methods have been
devised to detect ICs, several of which have been evaluated
for their potential for monitoring ICs in cancer patients
(Lambert et al., 1978). Some techniques depend on complement fixation, an indirect means of IC ascertainment, while
others measure ICs independent of this phenomenon. Of
potential interest in regard to early indirect detection
of tumors is a method of quantitating ICs using radiolabeled
Clq, part of the first component of complement.

In this assay, ^{125}I-labeled Clq is incubated with test sera that have been preincubated with EDTA to inactivate endogenous complement. Polyethylene glycol (PEG) is then added to the solution to selectively precipitate ICs so that any bound Clq, after centriguation, can be counted in a gamma-spectrometer (Zubler et al., 1976).

Clq-binding activity values have been reported to be significantly higher in the sera of cancer patients than in those of controls (Rossen et al., 1977; Höffken et al., 1977; Baldwin and Robins, 1980; Mod et al., 1980; Papsidero et al., 1979; Carpentier et al., 1982). Rossen et al. (1977) found higher Clq levels in patients with a variety of advanced malignancies, including breast, colon, and lung cancer, leukemia, and lymphoma, than in healthy blood bank donors. Papsidero et al. (1979) reported similar results in a study of women with breast cancer, fibrocystic disease of the breast, and healthy controls. The mean Clq-binding activity in women with breast cancer was about four times that of the controls, and approximately twice that of the patients with fibrocystic disease. Baldwin and Robins (1980) found that elevated Clq-binding activity could be used to distinguish patients with early breast cancer from people with fibrocystic disease, but only if heparin was added to the test sera. Carpentier et al. (1982) reported increased Clq-binding activity in 70% of 112 patients at the time of diagnosis of acute myeloid leukemia. The presence of ICs at diagnosis carried a poor prognosis.

Another recent investigation reported small quantities of ICs in newly diagnosed lung cancer patients (Guy et al., 1981). Sera from 80 patients with lung cancer, 20 patients with bronchitis, and 120 healthy controls were examined for ICs using both complement-dependent and complement-independent techniques capable of detecting different subspecies of ICs. Neither the solid- nor liquid-phase Clq-binding assays detected any significant differences in the prevalence of ICs between bronchitis patients and healthy controls, with a maximum of 15% of lung cancer patients having measurable ICs.

That these results differed dramatically from those of Rossen et al. (1977) may be attributed in part to the fact that patients of the former were newly diagnosed and less likely to have been carrying as large a tumor burden as patients in Rossen's study, all of whom had undergone surgical tumor resection. (In the study by Carpentier et al., however, the leukemia patients with elevated levels of ICs were also newly diagnosed.) Differences in the protocols of the IC assays may also partially explain the discrepancy. Finally, the heterogeneity of ICs with respect to relative proportions of antibody to antigen, as well as the kinds of antigens and classes and biologic activities of antibodies, may also contribute to these disparate results (see below).

Clq-binding activity may be valuable in the early detection of animal tumors in cancer bioassays. It is technically straightforward and relatively inexpensive. Höffken et al. (1978a,b), using a modification of the Clq assay described above, reported some interesting results of sequential monitoring of chemically induced tumors in rats. Subcutaneous, intraperitoneal, and pulmonary tumors were introduced by implantation or injection into syngeneic WAB/Not rats. The tumors were derived from hepatomas and a sarcoma originally induced by the oral administration of 4-dimethylaminoazo- benzene and 3-methylcholanthrene, respectively. When the tumor inoculum was 10^5 cells or greater, the investigators observed an initial peak of Clq-binding activity in rat sera, followed by a gradual decline to levels lower than normal. This decrease was attributed to a readily demon- strable antitumor antibody excess, in the presence of which IC cannot be quantitated without additional fractionation and separation (Nydegger et al., 1974).

This hypothesis was supported by subsequent measurements of ICs and antibodies in gel-filtration fractionated sera from rats bearing intraperitoneally implanted hepatomas (Höffken et al., 1978b). ICs were detected at early and late stages in fractionated sera, while Clq-binding activity measured in unfractionated sera declined despite progressive tumor growth. The authors concluded that

> ...it appears that the accurate quantitation of circulating immune complexes at late stages of tumour growth may be impeded by the development of antibody in excess and also by the induction of non-complement fixing tumour-specific IgG_2 antibodies, coupled with a reduction in levels of complement-fixing immunoglobulin of the IgG_1 subclass.

This implies that while Clq-binding activity may provide an early indication of tumor growth, it probably cannot be used to monitor tumor growth during the evolution of antibody excess and of noncomplement-fixing antibodies. However, a combination of this complement-dependent assay with one or more assays that do not depend on complement could be used to monitor tumor progression.

Because ICs differ not only in their ability to fix complement, but also in size, antigen content, antibody-antigen ratio, and antigenic class, a composite assay for diagnostic purposes has much to recommend it. An example of this is provided by Johny et al. (1981), who found that a composite method using three PEG-dependent techniques for IC detection compared favorably in sensitivity and specificity to the more complex Raji cell assay. Although these investigators were looking at ICs in various nonmalignant diseases, their findings regarding the characteristics of these tests can be applied to malignant states. The parallel use of multiple PEG-dependent markers with different specificities for antibody class and complement carries the following advantages:

> The techniques are relatively easy to perform and large numbers of samples may be handled simultaneously. Reagents are prepared by well-established methods and may be stored for long periods without decay. Less than 0.5 ml of serum is needed for duplicate determinations. [This composite method also] improves the likelihood that the material detected is immune complex [and reduces] the false positives and negatives associated with individual assays (Johny et al., 1981).

This composite index (C1q-binding activity, C1q solubility, and complement consumption assays) detected elevated levels of ICs in 88% of 32 serially tested leukemia patients (Mod et al., 1980). IC levels fluctuated independently of clinical findings, and the ICs measured by the different tests showed different patterns of fluctuation. These investigators inferred from their observations that the composition and structure of ICs evolves during the course of disease; the changes in ICs could involve different quantities and qualities both of tumor-related antigens (e.g., antigen excess, surface and nuclear antigens) and of antibodies (e.g., ability to fix complement, class, and subclass). This evolution is complex and dynamic, and monitoring it probably requires a composite battery of assays.

Several limitations of the usefulness of the C1q-binding

activity assay warrant further investigation. Some tumors shed antigens into the bloodstream, but it is not known whether the ICs measured by this assay are tumor-specific. Experimental results related to this question are inconsistent. Höffken et al. (1978b) reported finding complement-fixing and noncomplement-fixing tumor-specific antibodies in animals with chemically induced neoplasms. More recently, Guy et al. (1981) reported that they were unable to detect IC components unique to lung cancer patients with gel-filtration chromatography and polyacrylamide-gel electrophoresis of sera from lung cancer patients and others.

Circulating ICs are found in a variety of inflammatory, infectious, and autoimmune diseases, the presence of which could generate false-positive results in IC assays. These confounding conditions would present much less of a problem in animal bioassays than they do clinically. Still, it would be useful to be able to distinguish malignancy-related ICs from those found in other conditions. However, ICs measured by C1q-binding activity have not been well-characterized, and the assay itself has not been standardized.

Rossen et al. (1977) reported that with sucrose-density-gradient centrifugation, the C1q-binding activity in cancer patients' sera had sedimentation constants between 9S and 19S, while that for the sera of two patients with rheumatoid arthritis and 16 patients with IC glomerulonephritis had constants greater than 19S. Thus, the ICs in cancer patients were probably of lower molecular weight than those found in patients with autoimmune disease, which is consistent with the relative infrequency of IC symptoms in cancer patients. However, Gropp et al. (1980) reported that C1q-reactive ICs in 100 lung cancer patients sedimented between 19S and 30S in sucrose-density-gradient centrifugation. Thus the size, structure, and evolution of ICs need further experimental clarification.

Another potentially significant limitation is that C1q-binding activity decreases in the presence of excess antigen (Höffken et al., 1977), so massive antigen shedding from a large tumor burden could be masked by low C1q activity. This should not be a major impediment in an animal bioassay, however, because serial C1q assays would presumably detect an early increase in C1q-binding activity before extensive tumor growth.

CARCINOEMBRYONIC ANTIGEN (CEA)

Carcinoembryonic antigen (CEA) was one of the earliest
reported potential cancer markers. Its utility as an early
marker has not served that purpose effectively. The experience with CEA has been extensively reviewed (Fuks et al.,
1980; McIntire and Greenberg, 1981; Shively and Toss, 1980).
Lack of specificity and high incidences of both false-
positive and false-negative findings of circulating CEA
values render it a questionable marker of early neoplastic
activity.

Animal Studies

No extensive animal studies with CEA were found in the
literature, but CEA's continued expression in the blood of
the animal recipient of transplanted human cancer has been
documented (Goldberg and Hansen, 1972).

Human Studies

CEA has been used mainly in clinical medicine; sequential
measurements of its level in the blood detecting changes
in the clinical status of patients under treatment. CEA
has not been especially useful for screening asymptomatic
populations or for establishing a positive diagnosis of
cancer. There are no records of specific chemical agents
that have elicited measureable, increased circulating CEA
levels, but McCartney and Hoffer (1974) reported variously
increased levels in the blood of presumably healthy cigarette smokers. Increased levels have been reported in presumably normal human beings, in some patients with benign
neoplasms (LoGerfo et al., 1979), and in 15 to 20% of
patients with inflammatory disorders (pulmonary infections,
liver disease, pancreatitis, ulcerative colitis, and Crohn's
disease) that had no evidence of cancer (Constanza et al.,
1974). It is clear that the inability of the available
assay systems to distinguish among CEA levels from subjects
with localized malignant and benign tumors or from cigarette
smokers renders the CEA assay inadequate as an early predictor of neoplastic disease.

The available assay systems (Sizaret and Esteve, 1980) cannot distinguish among groups within a population that will
or will not develop CEA-producing malignant tumors. An
increased circulating CEA level alone is not diagnostic of
cancer. Levels 5 to 10 times greater than the upper limit

of the normal range established for a particular laboratory
(or assay system) should be considered strongly suggestive
of cancer in a patient and invite the use of further diagnostic methods (Fritschle et al., 1980; Kollman and Brennan,
1979). Among cancer patients, such increments are likely
to be associated with cancers of the pancreas (Holyoke et
al., 1979), ovary (Samaan et al., 1976), lung (Maxim et al.,
1981), heart, liver (Kojima et al., 1979), breast (Waalkes
and Tormey, 1978), and thyroid (Cimitan et al., 1979).

CEA levels are clinically informative in assessing the stage
and prognosis of a previously diagnosed tumor. Such inter-
pretations are made with caution because rising circulating
CEA levels do not necessarily indicate progression of the
disease. Nor can CEA values in the normal range be taken as
reliable indicators of localization or remission of disease.
Between 15 and 20% of patients with diagnosed cancers did
not show increased levels of circulating CEA (McIntire and
Greenberg, 1981).

Patients with colorectal or bronchial carcinomas have a
better record of survival when their preoperative levels
of circulating CEA are less than five times the normal
values (McIntire and Greenberg, 1981). The most efficacious
use of circulating CEA is in the sequential monitoring of
patients who have had surgery for colorectal cancer (Pompecki and Winkler, 1980). After completely successful
surgical removal of colorectal cancers, circulating CEA
levels returned to normal. The presence of residual tumor
correlated well with elevated postoperative values. Slow
postoperative elevations in CEA levels indicated local
recurrence, and rapid rises indicated hepatic and osseous
metastases (Chu et al., 1976).

The changing CEA levels and attendant changes in tumor
burden may reflect the efficacy of therapy; a continued
increase in circulating CEA indicates poor therapeutic
response. Also, smoking and intercurrent infections obscure
the clinical assessment of stable tumors (McIntire and
Greenberg, 1981).

Future research with CEA as a cancer marker should include
(1) the development of increased organ specificity of the
assay system (possibly through the use of monoclonal antibody technology), (2) the development of standards and
quality control systems for laboratories, and (3) the
development of panels of other cancer markers to be used
in combination with CEA.

IMMUNOLOGIC MARKERS IN MALIGNANT LYMPHOID TISSUES

Neoplasms of the immune system can be classified into four
main categories--lymphocytic leukemias, malignant lymphomas,
monocytic leukemias, and malignant histiocytoses--based on
the cell of origin (Lukes and Collins, 1975). Although the
search for antigens or markers that are specific for these
neoplasms has been going on for many years, little or no
solid evidence of their existence has been demonstrated.
Some markers that have been detected in the lymphoid tumors
are also found in normal tissues. This situation is encoun-
tered frequently, especially as more sensitive techniques
for antigen detection are developed. Nevertheless, one
cannot exclude the possibility that true markers are developed during tumorigenesis that are not detected by present
biochemical and immunologic techniques.

The following markers are frequently discussed in the
literature dealing with neoplasms of the immune system.
Whereas these markers are useful for determining the type
of cancer in patients or in animals, none is useful for
early diagnosis.

(1)   Erythrocyte rosette receptor. This marker may
facilitate the classification of acute lymphoblastic leukemia (ALL) into subtypes (T- or B-origin,
Bowman et al., 1981). It is found on T-lymphocyte
surfaces, both normal and neoplastic, and therefore has little value for diagnosis or prognosis.

(2)   Surface immunoglobulin. This marker is found pre-
dominantly on B-lymphocyte cell surfaces (Unanue
et al., 1971). Both normal and neoplastic B-cells
possess this surface marker (Fu et al., 1974; Rowe
et al., 1973), so that it has no diagnostic value.

(3)   Cytoplasmic immunoglobulin M (Preud'Homme and
Seligmann, 1974), Fc receptor (Moretta et al.,
1980; Pichler and Broder, 1978; Huber et al.,
1969), complement receptor (Reynolds et al.,
1975). These markers are found in normal lymphocytes and monocytes and are not applicable to
early tumor diagnosis.

(4)   Lymphocyte differentiation markers (Thy 1, Lyt,
Lyb, TL, Ia antigens). These markers are found on
normal lymphocytes during differentiation and are
not applicable to early tumor diagnosis (Panfili,
1980).

(5) HLA (histocompatibility) antigens. These markers
are human transplantation antigens found on normal
tissues and peripheral blood cells. When HLA typing was performed on a large number of cancer
patients, a very high incidence of cancer was
found in members belonging to the HL-A2 and HL-A12
types, but more screening must be performed before
conclusions relative to cancer can be made (Lloyd
et al., 1981; Lynch et al., 1975).

Recently, a subpopulation of circulating T-lymphocytes bearing surface ferritin was found in patients with breast cancer and untreated Hodgkin's disease (Giler and Moroz, 1978).
No such lymphocytes were demonstrated in normal individuals
or patients with benign breast disease. The appearance of
such a subpopulation in the circulation is thought to be a
manifestation of the neoplastic diseases. The identification of such T-lymphocytes may provide a tool for potential
diagnostic and prognostic use in the management of Hodgkin's
disease and breast cancer.

TUMOR-ASSOCIATED ANTIGENS (LESS AFP AND CEA)

Tumor-associated antigens are proteins that have been
detected by a number of methods to be present in established
tumors. Many of these antigens have been found in tumors of
a variety of tissues such as bowel, breast, cervix, brain,
ovary, liver, lung, and bone. The antigenic proteins have
been characterized in some instances and appear to be either
fetal proteins or proteins altered somehow in the cancerous
state.

Specific immunogenic tumor proteins have been detected in
the colon and pancreas of experimental animals with chemically induced tumors. An antigenic oncofetal protein was
found in a small-bowel adenocarcinoma of the rat--induced by
X-rays. It was common to 100 other radiation-induced rat
neoplasms (sites not specified), 12 colonic adenomas induced
by dimethylhydrazine, and 8 pancreatic adenomas induced by
dimethylbenzanthracene in the rat (Stevans et al., 1981).
Detection was by antiserum to the X-ray-induced adenocarcinoma against cell homogenates of the other neoplasms using
Ouchterlony plates. Tests using normal adult tissues were
consistently negative. The antigen was found in both the
tumor and the serum, but no tests were done during the

preneoplastic state. Other reports indicate that cross-reactive, tumor-specific antigens, such as those cited in the preceding reference, are not detectable in syngeneic hosts (Belnap et al., 1979). Cross-reactive, tumor-associated antigens in dimethylhydrazine- and nitroso-guanidine-induced colon tumors (not found in normal colon) have been demonstrated in the rat by Steele and Sjögren (1974). Cell-surface antigens have been detected also in methylcholanthrene-induced sarcomas in mice (De Leo et al., 1980).

Any carcinogen screening system using animals would be improved in time and cost if tumor-associated antigens could be detected before overt tumor formation. However, little is known about antigenic proteins in preneoplastic cells. Nevertheless, a few reports of animal models have indicated that specific antigenic proteins do exist in developing tumors. One concerns a chromosomal, nonhistone protein-DNA complex that induces antibodies that react with colon cells of the rats treated with dimethylhydrazine once per week for four weeks (Chiu et al., 1980). The antigen becomes detectable before histologic evidence of dysplasia or neoplasia is evident in the colon. The antibodies to this antigen do not react with either normal colon cells or hepatoma cells.

Other evidence that tumor-specific antigens may be found in the preneoplastic stage is suggested by the presence of tumor-specific antigens on rat liver cells transformed in vitro by each of two known carcinogens, dimethylnitrosamine and N-methyl-N'nitro-N-nitrosoguanidine (Yokota et al., 1979). The tumor-specific antigens were not present on normal or nonmalignant cells.

Such results lend some credence to the usefulness of tumor-associated antigens as tumor markers in a carcinogenicity screening test in animals and support the pursuit of intensified research.

Tumor-associated antigens have been found in a large number of human cancers. They have been detected in (1) breast tumors (Black et al., 1976; Springer et al., 1982; Hollins-head et al., 1974; Herberman, 1978) and sera from breast cancer patients (Lerner et al., 1978; Gorsky and Sulitzeanu, 1975), (2) benign breast lesions (Thomson et al., 1979), (3) cervical carcinomas (Haines et al., 1981), (4) brain tumors (Coakham et al., 1980), (5) ovarian tumors (Nishida et al., 1981), (6) the ovarian cystadenocarcinoma-associated antigen (Bhattacharya and Barlow, 1979; Lloyd, 1980; Imamura et al., 1978), (7) bone tumors (Hadley and Sindelar, 1979), and (8) lung tumors (Bell and Seetharam, 1979). Human antigenic "markers" have been reviewed also by Dodson and Menon (1979). The possibility of finding specific antigens in these and other types of tumors should be investigated in animal systems using the many carcinogens that have known tissue target sites. The procedure should include serial examination of target organs during the development of tumors to establish whether the marker is expressed in the "preneoplastic state." Controls using similar noncarcinogenic chemicals must be included.

The disadvantages of employing tumor-specific antigens as markers for carcinogenicity are apparent, also. Most have been associated with overt cancer and may not detect early or preneoplastic states. They are often tumor-tissue-specific, implying the need to anticipate the tissue(s) likely to be affected by a chemical in a screening program. Antigens that are specific for individual tumors may be of little or no use. The methods used for these immune tests vary from simple Ouchterlony antigen precipitation and complement-fixation to more complex ^{51}Cr-label release, lymphocyte migration, and other, more costly tests. No one method is applicable to all antigenic types, so that several may be required to detect protein changes in a screening mode. Last, we do not know the magnitude of false-positive or false-negative results that are likely to arise.

There are distinct advantages, on the other hand, in using immunologic methods for carcinogenic screening. Some methods are very sensitive and relatively simple and can ultimately be standardized and "packaged" for routine use, as is the case with the radioimmune assay. Such feasible immunologic assays need to be developed further for systems that show promise.

INADEQUATELY TESTED IMMUNOLOGIC MARKERS

Several potential immunologic markers were evaluated but were judged to be insufficiently tested for recognizing carcinognesis at this time.

Tumor Cell Antigens

Many reports were descriptive of diagnostic identification of specific tumor cells or tissues. These assays are useful as clinical tools rather than as markers of carcinogenesis in animals. In most cases there are no data on the sensitivity of detection or on the temporal relationship between the levels of these antigens in patient serum or urine and tumor burden or recurrence of tumors. No animal studies or correlations with nonclinical studies were found.

Assays found in the literature included those for the following antigens:

- Leukemic cell antigens (Greaves et al., 1975; Kersey et al., 1981; Reinherz et al., 1979).

- Breast tissue-associated antigen (Koestler et al., 1981; Ohno et al., 1979; Sloane et al., 1980; O'Brien et al., 1980; Nordquist et al., 1978; Black et al., 1976; Hollinshead et al., 1974).

- Melanoma antigen (Irie et al., 1976; Hollinshead, 1975).

- Lung tumor antigen (Coombes et al., 1978; Veltri et al., 1977; Bell and Seetharam, 1976,1979).

- Gastrointestinal and colorectal tumor antigens (Hakomori et al., 1977; Bara et al., 1978; Belnap et al., 1979).

- Tumor polypeptide antigen (Nemoto et al., 1979; Schwartz, 1976).

- T-antigen (Scheiffarth, 1979).

- Human sarcoma antigen (Sethi and Hirshaut, 1981).

- Hepatic antigens (Oon and Lan, 1979; Yokota et al., 1979).

Diagnostic Techniques

Tumor cells or tumor-associated antigens can be identified using markers from various assay systems. The assay markers per se may not be able to recognize carcinogenesis. In addition, insufficient data were found to substantiate strong correlations between assays and tumor burden or early tumorigenesis in human or animal subjects. The following techniques deserve further study and include assays of:

- Leukocyte migration inhibition (McCoy et al., 1976; Bubenik et al., 1981; McCoy et al., 1978).

- Labeling index (Barthold, 1981).

- Growth of tumor cells (Montesano et al., 1980; Hutter et al., 1978; Bubenikova et al., 1980).

- Erythrocyte sedimentation rate (Wolf et al., 1979; Thynne and Grening, 1980; Thynne, 1979; DeYoung et al., 1980; Jacobi, 1979).

- Electrophoretic mobility (Lewkonia et al., 1974; Hoffman et al., 1981a,1981b; Moser et al., 1980; Bubenik et al., 1981).

Some of these potential markers are treated in greater detail elsewhere in this review.

Changes in Components of the Immune Systems

Alteration of the levels of immunoglobulins (IgG, IgM, IgA), α_2-macroglobulin, complement components, or other components of the immune system in tumor-bearing animals or human patients have been described. There was little correlation between these changes and tumorigenesis or tumor burden, and no definition of specificity and sensitivity of the observed changes, so the following markers were deemed to require further development for use as early markers in carcinogenesis screening programs.

- Immunoglobulins (Pulay and Csömör, 1979; Rognum et al., 1980; Roberts et al., 1975; Solomon, 1980; Betkerur et al., 1980a,1980b).

- Macroglobulins, complement (Pulay and Csömör, 1979; Maxim et al., 1981; Sarjadi et al., 1980).

- Lymphocyte activation (Sjögren and Steele, 1975; Autio et al., 1979).

XIII

Miscellaneous Cancer Markers

R.A. Howd, E.F. Meierhenry, R.H. Suva

MISCELLANEOUS INDICATORS OF EXPERIMENTAL CARCINOGENESIS

The following suggested markers do not fit well in the foregoing categories but have been examined for their potential
as early indicators of carcinogenesis.

Ferritins

Ferritins are a group of proteins having an important function in iron storage and metabolism and are found in high
concentrations in the liver, spleen, and bone marrow (Giler
and Moroz, 1978). Acidic isoferritins are found in human
fetal liver and in primary lung, mammary, gastric, and
pancreatic carcinomas; they are called carcinofetal ferritins (Giler and Moroz, 1978; Maxim et al., 1981; Alpert et
al., 1979). Ferritin isolated from malignant tissue differs
electrophoretically from normal ferritin, but the molecular
basis for this is not known (Alpert et al., 1979). Elevated levels of such serum ferritin were found in patients
with various malignant diseases such as Hodgkin's disease;
chronic myeloblastic, granulocytic, and lymphatic leukemias;
myeloblastosis; breast cancer; multiple myeloma; malignant
lymphoma; carcinoma of the gastrointestinal tract; and germinal cell tumors of the testes (Marcus and Zinberg, 1975;
Tormey et al., 1979; Coombes et al., 1977; Order and Klein,
1980; Giler and Moroz, 1978; Jibiki et al., 1980). Elevated
levels of ferritin in serum have been found in 39 to 88%
of patients with the above malignancies (Tormey et al.,
1979; Coombes et al., 1977). One area of special interest
is the detection of patients with recurrent or metastatic

breast cancer. Studies have shown that 67 to 88% of these individuals have elevated serum levels of ferritin (Marcus and Zinberg, 1975; Coombes et al., 1977). However, serum ferritin levels are also increased in such nonmalignant conditions as hepatitis, cirrhosis, gastrointestinal ulceration (Marcus and Zinberg, 1975), hematologic disorders and after blood transfusion (Jibiki et al., 1980). Thus, the presence of these conditions would interfere with the specificity of diagnosis.

Recently, a subpopulation of circulating T-lymphocytes bearing surface ferritin was found in patients with breast cancer and untreated Hodgkin's disease (Giler and Moroz, 1978; Giler et al., 1979). No such lymphocytes were demonstrated in normal humans or in patients with benign breast disease. In one study, 45 of 47 patients with stage I or II carcinoma of the breast had ferritin-laden circulating T-lymphocytes (Giler et al., 1979).

Such a subpopulation in the circulation appears to be an early manifestation of certain neoplastic diseases, and its identification may provide a tool of potential diagnostic and prognostic importance in the management of Hodgkin's disease and breast cancer (Giler and Moroz, 1978).

In one animal study involving a comparison of ferritins in normal and malignant rat liver and kidney, it was determined that ferritins from tumors migrated faster electrophoretically and had a lower antibody-binding capacity than did ferritins from normal tissue (Linder and Munro, 1973).

Additional study of tumor ferritins and ferritin-bearing T-lymphocytes in laboratory animals appears warranted.

Hydroxyproline

Hydroxyproline, an amino acid found in collagen but not in other proteins, has been studied as a marker of metastasis of cancer to bone. It is apparently synthesized in situ and incorporated into the macromolecular collagen precursor; dietary hydroxyproline is not used in collagen synthesis by the rodent (Harper, 1969). Normal collagen turnover in bones, tendons, and other tissues results in the release of hydroxyproline, some of which is excreted into the urine intact or as a component of small peptides (Becker et al., 1976). Urinary hydroxyproline can thus be used as an index of the collagen turnover rate, although it is complicated by

the concomitant excretion of dietary hydroxyproline. In
some clinical studies, the assay of urinary hydroxyproline
had been preceded by two days of administration of a low-
hydroxyproline diet. For animal studies such dietary
control would not be required if chow with protein from
nonanimal sources were used exclusively. Then the determination of urinary hydroxyproline would be a simple means
of following metastases of tumors to bone in screening for
carcinogens.

Only human studies were found to be reported in our literature survey. We presume that the technique should work in
laboratory animals, although hydroxyproline biochemistry
appears to be somewhat species-dependent. In humans, for
example, 4-hydroxyproline is the form of the amino acid in
collagen, whereas in rats 3-hydroxyproline also is a component of tail collagen (Harper, 1969). All the reports of
cancer markers refer to the assay of urinary hydroxyproline
or hydroxyproline-containing peptides, without mention of
blood levels. However, hydroxyproline can be detected free
in serum and in small-peptide fractions (Arnold et al.,
1969).

Hydroxyproline is commonly analyzed by acid hydrolysis of
peptides, then oxidation to a pyrolle, reaction with p-
dimethylaminobenzaldehyde, and assay by spectrophotometry
(Henry et al., 1974). An autoanalyzer technique is also
available (Becker et al., 1976).

Disease of bone formation or its destruction can give false
positive results in humans (Paget's disease, for example),
although such complications would be much less likely in
a controlled animal population. In humans, a significant
rise in urinary hydroxyproline appears to be a more sensitive detector of bone metastases than is radiologic scanning
(Szymanovicz et al., 1980). The sensitivity of this urinary
assay as a measure of tumor mass has not been evaluated in
animals.

One cogent question remains--would it be useful to obtain
such information in an animal study? If one is merely
screening for the carcinogenic potential of a compound, and
other tests failed to disclose a primary tumor, detection
of bone metastases would be valuable. For animal testing
of the efficacy of a multiple cancer marker screen, it might
be desirable to include a urinary hydroxyproline assay at
an initial stage to reveal the presence of tumors that other

markers may have missed. If other markers are found to be adequate, the hydroxyproline test could be eliminated.

Mallory Bodies

Mallory bodies are abnormal cytoplasmic structures that have been observed in the hepatocytes of human patients with alcoholic cirrhosis, hepatocellular carcinoma, and various other hepatic disorders (Denk et al., 1979; Meierhenry et al., 1981). These inclusions have also been seen in alveolar epithelial cells of the lung in patients with asbestosis, radiation pneumonitis, and nonspecific conditions (Warnock et al., 1980). Mallory body-type inclusions also occur in hepatocellular carcinomas in mice exposed to the carcinogens dieldrin (Meierhenry et al., 1981) and griseofulvin (Denk et al., 1979) and in hepatocytes cultured from carcinomas produced in rats by the carcinogen diethylnitrosamine (Borenfreund et al., 1980; Borenfreund and Bendich, 1978).

Mallory bodies are composed of tangled masses of filaments, related to intermediate-size filaments, which are part of the cytoskeleton (Meierhenry et al., 1981; Denk et al., 1979). Disruption of the filaments may interfere with the orderly flow of information between the cell plasma membrane and the nucleus (Borenfreund et al., 1980; Borenfreund and Bendich, 1978). Additionally, it has been speculated that an accumulation of intermediate-size filaments could either induce or result from an oncogenic transformation (Trump et al., 1980; Borenfreund et al., 1980).

Because Mallory body-type changes are induced rapidly in hepatocytes after exposure to two carcinogens (12 weeks in mice fed griseofulvin and 10 weeks in rats given diethylnitrosamine) and are present in three potentially preneoplastic conditions in humans (asbestosis, radiation pneumonitis, and alcoholic cirrhosis), additional investigation of their potential as an early in vivo marker of carcinogenicity is warranted.

Polyamines

The polyamines putrescine, spermidine, and spermine play important roles in cellular growth and proliferation (Canellakis et al., 1979). Their levels (and the levels of their synthetic enzymes in tissues) could be expected to rise with the increased cell growth found in rapidly growing tumors. These compounds have been extensively studied in recent years as potential tumor markers in a wide variety of clinical conditions, in experimental animals with chemically induced or transplantable tumors, and in cell culture systems (Bohuon and Assicot, 1976; Russell, 1977; Jänne et al., 1978; Russell, 1978; Canellakis et al., 1979; Nagarajan and Sukumar, 1979; Russell and Durie, 1979; Marton et al., 1981; Wasserstrom et al., 1981). Polyamine concentrations have been measured in tissues (correlated with the rate of cell growth), in plasma, whole blood, cerebrospinal fluid, urine, and tissue culture media. In nearly all such investigations, increases in one or more of the polyamines (usually putrescine, sometimes spermidine, rarely spermine) have been found to correlate with cancer growth. Increases in the activity of the polyamine synthetic enzyme ornithine decarboxylase and the catabolic enzyme diamine oxidase are also correlated with changes in polyamine synthesis and release into extracellular fluids in rapid tissue growth (Kallio et al., 1977; Scalabrino et al., 1978; Costa et al., 1979; Herzfeld and Greengard, 1980; Matsui et al., 1980; Matsushima and Bryan, 1980; Olson and Russell, 1980; Webber et al., 1980; Sessa et al., 1981; Scalabrino et al. 1981; Van Wijk et al., 1981).

The results of some of the earlier polyamine studies may not be reliable because of the limitations of the analytical methods, particularly for the low levels of polyamines in serum. Most of the polyamines in blood exist in erythrocytes (RBCs) in a free (nonconjugated) form at concentrations high enough for simple analysis by modern analytical methods (Savory et al., 1979; Desser et al., 1980a,b; Shipe et al., 1980; Takami and Nishioka, 1980; Uehara et al., 1980). The RBCs apparently accumulate polyamines from the serum and effectively provide an index of time-averaged polyamine release from tissues, which may eliminate misleading short-term spikes in polyamine levels (Takami et al., 1979).

Polyamines are conjugated in the liver before being excreted into the urine. Urinary polyamines are commonly analyzed after acid hydrolysis of these conjugates. Urine is the most available fluid for polyamine analysis, has reasonably high polyamine levels, and requires a noninvasive method of sampling.

The numerous studies of polyamines in humans and animals allow the utility and shortcomings of polyamine analysis as a marker for experimental carcinogenesis to be relatively well defined.

First, all cells require and produce polyamines at a rate related to that of cell growth. However, there may be differences in the rate of polyamine production and release into the extracellular space among different cell types that are independent of the rate of cell growth. Second, not all invasive tumors grow rapidly; on the contrary, an animal marker for tumorigenesis may be more useful when tumor development is very slow. Thus a positive marker assay could allow sacrifice of test animals for in situ tumor confirmation long before palpable or life-threatening tumors are evident. Third, treatments, diseases, or life stages (e.g., pregnancy) causing rapid growth of tissues also result in elevated polyamines. For these reasons, polyamine assays as clinical cancer markers have been plagued with high false-negative and false-positive rates. In experimental studies, the same factors apply, but the use of a more homogenous, controlled population should decrease the random differences in polyamine levels. However, drug or chemical treatments causing tissue damage and repair, or growth stimulation, might generate false-positive results.

In rodents with transplanted or chemically induced tumors, urinary putrescine concentrations correlated well with tumor burden (Fujita et al., 1976,1978; Anehus et al., 1981); about a 2-cm^3 tumor was required to produce a significant increase in the urinary putrescine excretion rate in rats (Anehus et al., 1981). Analysis of a specific conjugated polyamine, N^1-acetylspermidine, in the urine of tumor-implanted rats showed no significant increase until a tumor burden of about 35 g was reached (Seiler et al., 1981). This specific analysis appears to be unsuitable for early-marker studies. Increased RBC putrescine, spermidine, and spermine levels have been correlated with tumor burden in rodents with rapidly growing implanted tumors (Shipe et al., 1980; Takami and Nishioka, 1980; Uehara et al., 1980). In an interesting study on RBC polyamine levels in horses with very slowly growing (spontaneous) melanomas (Desser et al., 1980a), no increase in polyamines was detected despite increasing spread of the melanoma. The tumor burden was not clear from the data, and results were complicated by a falling polyamine RBC concentration with increasing age in this small subject population.

Striking clinical success in correlating brain tumor growth

with polyamine concentration in CSF has been reported, but
this would be of less interest for studies in rodents
because of the low incidence of chemically induced brain
tumors and the difficulty of obtaining adequate samples.
Assays of RBC (unconjugated) polyamines, urinary total polyamines, or urinary putrescine are the logical choices for
animal studies. Studies that we have reviewed have not compared the RBC and urinary polyamine assays for sensitivity
of tumor detection in an appropriate animal paradigm. In
the experiments of Fujita et al. (1976, 1978), mean levels
of urinary putrescine were significantly higher in treated
animals than in controls weeks before there were significant numbers of tumor-related deaths in rats and mice with
slowly developing chemically induced tumors. However, it
is not clear in the report of Fujita et al. (1976) whether
the increased urinary putrescine levels were the result of
increased tissue regeneration after toxic tissue damage from
repeated administration of a carcinogen or were products of
developing tumor(s). In their other study (Fujita et al.,
1978) the administration of a single subcutaneous dose of a
carcinogen made non-site-specific, noncancer effects much
less likely, and provides excellent support for the utility
of urinary putrescine as a "specific" marker under these
conditions.

Thus, the applicability of using urinary polyamines as a
marker in animal carcinogenesis has been demonstrated in
relevant animal systems. Whether RBC polyamine analysis
might be as sensitive and specific as urinary analysis is
unclear. Blood sampling is much quicker and cheaper than
urine collection, so it would theoretically be preferable
to use blood. Because increased polyamine levels represent
either increased rates of tissue growth or cell death, or
both, the analysis of these compounds does not provide a
unique marker for cancer. However, in combination with the
measurement of more specific marker substances, polyamine
analysis could have significant value as an indicator of
progressive deleterious effects of chemicals or treatments
in subacute or chronic studies.

Polyamine analysis is also useful as a marker in humans,
with the limitations described above for animals. In general, the tumor burden would be quite large before RBC or
urine polyamine levels would increase significantly. Nevertheless, polyamine analysis can provide evidence of large or
occult tumors, particularly when used as part of a multiple
marker screen (Russell and Durie, 1979). Also, polyamines

can aid in assessing tumor response to therapy because their
excretion tends to rise when tumor cells are dying (Russell,
1978; Russell and Durie, 1979; Nishioka et al., 1980).
Extracellular polyamine levels may also rise during recurrence of tumor growth after successful therapy, and thus
indicate relapse (Fulton et al., 1980; Marton, 1981; Marton
et al., 1981).

Resistance of Altered Hepatocyte Foci to Iron Accumulation

One method for detecting early hepatocyte foci in carcinogenicity bioassays has involved the administration of excess
iron to rats and mice before exposing them to N-2-fluorenyl-
acetamide (FAA) (Watanabe and Williams, 1978; Williams,
1980; Williams and Watanabe, 1978; Hirota and Williams,
1979), to mice before benzopyrene administration (Ohmori
et al., 1981), and to mice before the development of spontaneous hepatocellular tumors (Ohmori et al., 1981; Williams
et al., 1979).   In these studies, all proliferative hepatocellular lesions at the various stages of development contained less iron than the surrounding liver.   These areas
were easily detected histochemically and generally corre-
sponded to areas of enzymatic alteration as revealed by
other methods (Ohmori et al., 1981; Williams, 1980; Hirota
and Williams, 1979).

Iron-resistant foci appeared within three to 13 weeks of
exposure to FAA (Williams, 1980; Williams and Watanabe,
1978), but after cessation of exposure, most foci reverted,
were able to accumulate iron, and could no longer be distinguished after 24 to 26 weeks (Watanabe and Williams, 1978;
Williams and Watanabe, 1978).   In the above experiments hun-
dreds of early foci per liver were detected.   However, if
other similarly treated animals were observed for 22 months,
often only one or two hepatocellular carcinomas per liver
developed.   Thus, it could not be determined that any particular focus would develop into hepatocellular carcinoma.

In summary, resistance to iron accumulation shows promise as
a marker of early hepatocellular focus-formation, although
the significance of the foci is yet to be determined.   Testing with many more carcinogens needs to be conducted before
a final appraisal can be made.

Seromucoid

Seromucoid (SMC) is a subfraction of α-globulin measured by
radioimmunoassay.   The serum level of SMC was consistently

elevated in rats fed benzenamine, 3'-methyl-4-dimethylamino-
benzene (3'-methyl DAB) (Odani et al., 1980), increasing
together with liver damage during the first three weeks of
feeding, with an elevation persisting steadily from six to
15 weeks. It appears that increased SMC synthesis occurs in
both benign and malignant liver tissue. Further experiments
are needed to determine whether other carcinogens elevate
SMC, whether liver toxins can be distinguished from liver
carcinogens, and whether other types of tumors also elevate
SMC.

64DP

A DNA binding protein that shows considerable promise as
a human cancer marker has been purified from human serum
(Katsunuma et al., 1980). Katsunuma et al. isolated this
protein (called 64DP), developed a radioimmunoassay, and
screened a large number of cancer patients. The protein
level was elevated in 84 of 87 patients, and in 8 of 8
"early" cancer patients, compared to both healthy controls
and those with nonmalignant disease.

The protein has not been examined in animals, but the
experience with humans suggests that a similar analysis of
DNA binding proteins in animals is warranted.

Zinc Glycinate Marker

In studies of human tissue using immunofluorescence microscopy, the zinc glycinate marker (ZGM) appeared to be quite
specific for gastrointestinal adenocarcinomas in 40 of 45
patients, whereas 22 of 22 non-gastrointestinal tumors were
negative (Saravis et al., 1978). Another report listed ZGM
as present in 26 of 29 colon carcinomas, but it was also
present in adjacent normal tissue in almost all patients
(Doos et al., 1978). In cell blocks from 25 cases of pleural or peritoneal effusions, 17 (68%) were positive for ZGM
(Saravis et al., 1978).

No animal data were available for evaluation.

MISCELLANEOUS COMPOUNDS WITH LIMITED OR UNKNOWN POTENTIAL AS CANCER MARKERS IN ANIMALS

Many other substances have been investigated as potential
markers in human cancer, but the data are too limited to
suggest applicability to animal studies. Some of the more

interesting ones are described below; others are summarized in Table XIII-1.

Abnormal Peptides

Abnormal peptides associated with tumors of the pancreas (Schwartz, 1979), lung (Szymanovicz et al., 1980), and other tissues have been described in humans, and may also be produced in animals, but no specific data are available.

Ornithine Metabolism

An increased rate of ornithine metabolism has been reported recently in cancer patients (Webber et al., 1980), probably related to the increased ornithine decarboxylase activity and enhanced polyamine synthesis in tumors. The measurement of this metabolic rate would be unlikely to be superior to polyamine assay.

Fibrin

Increased fibrin degradation products have been observed in the blood or urine of patients with various types of tumors (Haselager and Vreeken, 1981). Particularly with bladder cancer, increased fibrin in the urine may be expected—considering the generally enhanced fibrinolytic activity of tumor cells.

Catecholamine Metabolites

Patients with neuroblastoma may excrete large amounts of the catecholamine metabolites homovanillic acid and vanillactic acid and increased amounts of cystathionine (Covington et al., 1974; Laug et al., 1978). The incidence of this cancer in experimental animals is too low for analysis of these biochemicals to be of value in screening for carcinogenesis.

Bence-Jones Protein

Although it is diagnostic of multiple myeloma in humans, Bence-Jones protein is not promising as a cancer marker in animals. It is specific for malignant human plasma cells and appears after the disease is established (Nery and Neville, 1976; Tizard, 1977).

Casein

The blood level of casein, or of casein-like proteins, has been evaluated as a specific human cancer marker in several studies (Pich et al., 1976; Cowen et al., 1978; Rochman, 1978). It was initially presumed that finding elevated casein levels in the blood of nonlactating women would be a significant indication of abnormal cell growth, particularly of mammary tissue. However, most tumors, including most mammary tumors, do not produce casein levels significantly above background. Background levels arise from a low rate of production of casein-like proteins by many epithelial cells and exocrine glands (Pich et al., 1976). The low "positive" rate derives from a wide variety of tumor stem cells and dedifferentiated cells.

Measurement of casein in blood has been of little use diagnostically and has been largely abandoned. Its prospects for screening chemicals in animals are poor.

Globulins

In one study of azo-dye hepatic carcinogenesis in rats, α_1-globulin decreased early in the experiment (weeks 1 to 5); however, after tumors appeared, α_1-, α_2-, and β-globulins became elevated (Odani et al., 1980). This biphasic change in globulins would make their measurements for animal screening of little value.

Two studies indicated that α-globulins are generally elevated in patients with advanced ovarian cancer and are somewhat indicative of the clinical stage of the disease (Order and Klein, 1980; Order et al., 1979).

β_2-Microglobulin (Human)

Serum levels of β_2-microglobulin ($\beta_2 M$) in humans with various types of malignancies have not been an effective test for carcinogenesis (Coombes et al., 1977; Jibiki et al., 1980; Vladutin et al., 1981; Sarjadi et al., 1980; Cooper and Plesner, 1980; Staab et al., 1980; Kanoa et al., 1979; Johnson et al., 1980) not only because of a high rate of false negatives but because levels of $\beta_2 M$ are readily influenced by renal dysfunction (Cooper and Plesner, 1980). The following false negative rates were obtained: 44% in lung, liver, gall bladder, or pancreatic cancer (Jibiki et al., 1980); 54% in ovarian carcinoma (Sarjadi et al., 1980); 66% in bronchogenic carcinoma (Coombes et al., 1977); and 87% in testicular cancer (Johnson et al., 1980).

When $\beta_2 M$ was used as part of a battery of tests in patients with gynecologic malignancies (Sarjadi et al., 1980), 76%

of patients with cervical carcinoma had elevations of one or more of the following: $\beta_2 M$, lactate dehydrogenase, sialyltransferase, or spermine. In addition, 79% of patients with ovarian cancer had increases in $\beta_2 M$, sialyltransferase, carcinoembryonic antigen, or α-chain fetal hemoglobin.

It would appear that $\beta_2 M$ shows little promise as a solitary marker in humans. It apparently has not been evaluated in laboratory animal systems.

Melanoma-Specific Protein

A melanoma-specific protein (MSP) has been isolated from human urine and characterized (Bennett and Cooke, 1980). MSP is distinct from alpha-fetoprotein (AFP) and carcino-embryonic antigen (CEA), and does not appear to be fetal in origin. In advanced melanoma, MSP lacks the sialic acid groups found on the protein in early-stage patients. No statistics have been presented, so the predictive value of this marker cannot be established. It needs to be sought in melanomas of animals.

Pregnancy-Associated Macroglobulin

Pregnancy-associated macroglobulin (PAM) has apparently not been evaluated in animal systems, and it appears to be of limited value after extensive human studies (Anderson et al., 1976; Coombes et al., 1977, 1978, 1980; Dent and McCulloch, 1980; Malkin et al, 1978). Nevertheless, an equivalent search for a PAM-like protein should be pursued in several animal species.

Serum Copper

The rise in serum copper occurs late and has not been shown to predate the onset of cancer detectable by other means, making this an unlikely candidate for a predictive marker (Andrews, 1979; Jacobi, 1979; Linder et al., 1979; Volm et al., 1972; Wolf et al., 1979).

Table XIII-1

MARKERS JUDGED TO HAVE UNKNOWN OR LOW POTENTIAL
IN ANIMAL SCREENING SYSTEMS

Marker	Reason	References
Ectopic peptide	No data	Odell et al., 1977
Actin	Only histologic data	Gabbiani et al., 1975
Connective tissue activating protein	No correlation with cancer	Castor et al., 1981
Free secretory protein	Insufficient data	Order et al., 1975
Total urinary protein	Correlated only with advanced disease	Rudman et al., 1979
Amine metabolites	No correlation with cancer	Hansen et al., 1980
CSF lipids	No correlation with cancer	Hildebrand, 1973

(Continued)

Table XIII-1 (Continued)

Marker	Reason	References
Triglycerides	No correlation with cancer	Du et al., 1979
Gross cystic disease fluid protein	No correlation with cancer	Haagensen et al., 1978
Retinoic acid binding protein	Found only in cells	Rattanapanone et al., 1981
Lipoprotein X	Poor correlation with cancer	Rubies-Prat et al., 1976
Transferrin	Insufficient positive data	Kaneko et al., 1980; Pulay and Csömör, 1979
Thyroglobulin	Not promising in humans, no animal data	Rose, 1981
Plasma zinc	Insufficient data	Andrews, 1979
Plasminogen activator	No correlation with cancer transformation	Dolbeare et al., 1980; Montesano et al., 1980

(Continued)

Table XIII-1 (Concluded)

Marker	Reason	References
Lactoferrin	Insufficient data	Maxim et al., 1981
Haptoglobin	Limited data hold little promise	Coombes et al., 1977; Cowen et al., 1978; Odani et al., 1980
α_2-H-globin	Not specific to cancer	Tormey et al., 1979
Albumin and prealbumin	Insufficient positive data	Du et al., 1979, Feron and Kruysse, 1977; Gerber et al., 1981; Kaneko et al., 1980

XIV

Summary

G. Freeman

Several means are being used to improve the recognition
and control of biological processes that lead to cancer.
The commonplace approach has been through early evidence
of the clinical disease and a search for its associated
markers. More basic approaches include prevention and the
related scan for causative exogenous agents. A third major
approach, in its embryonic stage, offers impelling hope for
critical insights. It is the rapidly burgeoning research to
expose molecular genetic mechanisms that appear to determine
the neoplastic phenotypes of cells, their initiation, and
their markers. Such phenotypes may occur "spontaneously"
or may be the result of contact between potentially effective exogenous incitants and a vulnerable cytomolecular
milieu. Then, stepwise, either by point mutation (Tabin,
1982), translocation (Klein, 1981), or altered regulation
of genes, cells within a tissue are selected for continuous,
unruly replication (Logan and Cairns, 1982). Activation
of a normal growth gene (Goyette, 1983; Pearson, 1968) may
be an initial step in such a sequence, leading in time to
sustained growth.

Prevention and early detection of cancer are primary respon-
sibilities of private institutions and governmental environmental protection agencies, such as EPA, and are the
ultimate concern of this survey. The search for putative
markers of neoplastic growth has been intensive, with most
of the observations having been made through studies of
human disease. These studies have also provided a likely
source of markers that are sought in animal species that

are known or likely to be susceptible hosts for malignant neoplasms (Jones et al., 1978; Pollard et al., in press). Thus, animal models that can be used to distinguish onco- genic chemical agents from other agents that may pollute the environment are emphasized here.

This purview of putative cancer markers is concerned mainly with relatively short-term assays in laboratory animals. The kaleidoscopic spectrum of tests for markers of onco- genesis reported in the recent literature varies with the class of chemical compound being tested; route of adminis- tration of a chemical and its dosage regimen; nature and degree of toxicity; species of animal and its perinatal status, age, and sex; genetic strain; and accessory factors such as promotion, dietary management, partial excision of the liver, and thoroughness of pathologic examination.

The major advantage of an animal assay for oncogenesis is the access it allows to all tissues for disclosure of the initial site (target tissue) of neoplasia and the nature of toxicity to cells. Importantly, incidental complicating types of disease can be recognized and evaluated in rela- tion to the oncogenic process. Such studies in animals may enable better correlations to be made between morphology and reliable cancer markers in blood, urine, and serial biopsies and should improve specificity and sensitivity for detecting early neoplasia. Presumably, blood, urine, or tissue samples will have been obtained from both experi- mental and control animals at appropriate intervals prior to termination of the experiment for determination of physiologic, immunologic, biochemical, or morphologic changes indicative of the development of neoplasia. Many such markers, alone and in combination as profiles, have been evaluated for their ability to reveal the onset of cancer in animals and man.

Markers have been studied during the administration of numerous toxic chemicals. Some markers of convincing but not universal credibility provide both histochemical and biochemical evidence for neoplastic growth in the livers of rats and mice. Outstanding examples are GGT and AFP (see Chapters V and XII). Abnormal levels of these proteins can be detected by staining of focus-forming cells in tissue and can also be determined quantitatively in serum. Their levels tend to vary with time, related to the development of neoplasia. GGT- and AFP-identifiable foci or cells may form nodules that often have the capacity to develop into

primary hepatocarcinomas. However, the types of differentiation among GGT- and AFP-staining cells have not been
thoroughly established. Also, a deficiency in taking up
histochemically observable levels of Fe by the focal cells
and a reduction in some other enzyme activities detected
histochemically often accompany positive GGT-staining and
serve as supporting markers for putative neoplastic sites.

Other useful markers result from the effects of carcinogens
on DNA or RNA (see Chapters III and IV). Augmented DNA
polymerase activity is detected by the increased incorporation of tritiated thymidine, which reflects an abnormal
persistence of cellular replication. Abnormal patterns
of growth can often be differentiated during postmortem
examination from the nonspecific, compensatory changes due
to repair and growth following injury. DNA also may be
modified by adducts from exogenous test chemicals or their
metabolic products. Such unusually modified nucleosides and
bases may act as antigens against which specific antibodies
can be generated and used as markers. Transfer RNAs (tRNAs)
are abundantly methylated and otherwise modified by several
highly specific enzymes found in normal tissue. These modified residues can be detected in increased amounts in urine
of cancer-bearing animals. Elevated and disproportionate
amounts of such excreted, modified nucleosides from tRNAs
can be determined either by reverse-phase HPLC or by immunologic tests using specific antibodies.

The immune system can produce antibodies to abnormal cellular products of tumors (see Chapter XII). Oncogenic-
dependent immune complexes may thereby be generated and
measured in the serum. Complicating nononcogenic autoimmune
complexes may be distinguished by examining animals at
autopsy. Another immunologic marker resides in the LAI
test, in which monocytes, sequestered from an animal, are
examined for their natural capacity to adhere to glass
surfaces. An acquired property that inhibits such adherence
of macrophages is a marker for cancer and can be quantified.

In addition to the above most promising types of cancer
markers in animals, one or more of the following may be
included to advantage in establishing a battery of tests
for putative oncogenic markers. They are ODC and its associated polyamines (see Chapter XIII), galactosyl transferase
isoenzyme II (see Chapter VI), alkaline phosphatase (see
Chapter IX) and ferritin (see Chapter XIII), and their
respective isoenzymes. All are determined in blood, and

some polyamines can also be measured in urine. Other potentially useful markers that require more investigation are
epoxide hydrolase, glycosyl transferases, lipid-bound sialic
acid, and amylase (see text for their evaluations).

A prospectively planned, biological screening of the rapidly
growing store of compounds to be tested that would incorporate the numerous contributory biological variables and
designs may prove to be economically prohibitive. However,
if early temporal criteria for recognition of induction of
cancer were established, the search for associated markers
could be more securely directed at their specificity and
time of onset. Sensitivity could then be improved. Almost
all known and suspected compounds included in this review
are classified according to available evidence as "conclusive," "suggestive," or "indeterminate" inducers of cancer
among 2400 compounds in one compilation (Sax, 1981). It
would be remiss to ignore the enormous accumulation of
temporal and other data that await organization and digestion by computer analysis. Besides sources such as IARC
(1982), Sax (1981), and Tomatis (1979), several other data
bases can be used from which to concentrate and evaluate
significant variables for screening. Analysis of available
data would help to characterize separate variables, such as
type of compound, animal species target site, effective dose
regimen, route of administration, and, especially, duration
of the preneoplastic period. These quasi-quantitative and
qualitative backgrounds would lead to more efficient testing
and evaluation of markers. Such a procedure would be relatively economical and is likely to elicit a rich residue
of data with which to design tests for markers of chemical
oncogenesis in animals.

Another major step in scanning biological material for
cancer markers is the application of computer analysis to
two-dimensional electrophoresis of serum and other partially
purified biological materials (Westerbrink and Havsteen,
1982). This approach offers real promise for the potential
separation and identification of cancer-associated bio-
molecular species from both animals and man.

Many of the substances that have been reviewed in the text
as putative markers in man may well have several counterparts in experimental animals that are subjected to chemical
oncogenesis, such as relatively specific isoenzyme patterns.
Such isoenzymes need to be sought more agressively in blood,
urine, and tissues. Some may become detectable in the

general two-dimensional electrophoretic scanning being studied in several laboratories. Inconsistencies could then be resolved by the generation of highly specific monoclonal antibodies to cancer-associated isoenzymes.

Similary, excessive hormone production in animals may mimic those diseases in man that reflect the presence of hyperplastic and hyperactive endocrine tissues. It may be rewarding to develop a battery of tests to measure hormone levels in animals equivalent to those already explored in man.

Ultimately, it might become practical to organize a central library of tumor antigens from which specific antibodies would be generated for screening tissues and body fluids of experimental animals for markers.

In summary, the massive search for a practically acceptable, relatively short-term test in animals to identify exogenous oncogenic chemicals has thus far not provided readily useful and conclusive tests. However, many cancer markers appear promising, and newer knowledge continues to illuminate basic mechanisms of oncogenesis at the molecular level. Such information, combined with the development of more sensitive laboratory techniques, promises to result in their effective application for the early detection of markers in screening for chemical oncogenesis in animal studies. In time, the growing trend toward using nuclear magnetic resonance may apply to animal studies.

References

Abelev GI.   Production of embryonic serum alphaglobulin
by hepatomas.   Review of experimental and animal data.
Cancer Res 1968; 28:1344-1350

Abelev GI, Perova SD, Khramkova NI, Postnikova ZA, Irlin IS.
Production of embryonal α-globulin by transplantable mouse
hepatomas.   Transplantation 1963; 1:174-180

Adams WS, Davis F, Nakatoni M.   Purine and pyrimidine excretion in normal and leukemic subjects.   Am J Med 1960; 28:
726-734

Adams WS, Davis F, Nakatoni M.   Pseudouridine metabolism.
II. Urinary excretion in gout, psoriasis, leukemia and
heterozygous oroticaciduria.   Lab Clin Med 1962; 59:
852-858

Adinolfi M.   Human alpha-fetoprotein 1956-1978.   Adv Human
Genet 1979; 9:165-228

Agostini C, Secchi M, Venturelli D.   5'-Nucleotidase
activity in liver homogenates of rats treated with CCl_4,
colchicine, cyclohexamide, emetine, ethanol, ethionine,
and 5-fluorotryptophan.   Experientia 1980; 36:1067-1068

Alpert E, Quaroni A, Goldenberg DM.   Alteration in tryptic
peptide patterns of ferritins purified from human colon
carcinoma.   Biochim Biophys Acta 1979; 58:193-197

Alsabti EA, Muneir K.   Serum proteins in breast cancer.   Jpn
J Exp Med 1979; 59:235-240

Amador E, Zimmerman TS, Wacker WEC. Urinary alkaline phosphatase activity. I. Elevated urinary LDH and alkaline phosphatase activities for the diagnosis of renal adenocarcinomas. J Am Med Assoc 1963; 185:769-775

Anderson GR, Kovacik WP. LDH_k, an unusual oxygen-sensitive lactate dehydrogenase expressed in human cancer. Proc Nat Acad Sci USA 1981; 78:3209-3213

Anderson JM, Stimson WH, Gettinby G, Jhunjhunwala KK, Burt RW. Detection of mammary micrometastases by pregnancy-associated α_1-glycoprotein (PAG, α_2-PAG or PAM) and carcinoembryonic antigen (CEA). Eur J Cancer 1979; 15:709-714

Anderson JM, Stimson WH, Kelly F. Preclinical warning of recrudescent mammary cancers by pregnancy associated alpha macroglobulin. Br J Surg 1976; 63:819-822

Anderson T. Testicular germ cell neoplasms: Recent advances in diagnosis and therapy. Ann Intern Med 1979; 90:373-385

Andrews GS. Studies of plasma zinc, copper ceruloplasmin, and growth hormone with special reference to carcinoma of the bronchus. J Clin Pathol 1979; 32:329-333

Anehus S, Bengtsson G, Andresson G. Urinary putrescine and plasma lactate dehydrogenase as markers of experimental adenocarcinoma growth. Eur J Cancer 1981; 17:511-518

Anonymous. Categorization of carcinogens by mechanism meets consensus. Food Chem News 1982; 22:34-39

Armitstead PR, Gowland G. The leucocyte adherence inhibition test in cancer of the large bowel. Br J Cancer 1975; 32:568-573

Arnold E, Hvidberg E, Rasmussen S. Methodological studies of the distribution of hydroxyproline in human serum. Scand J Clin Lab Invest 1969; 24:231-235

Asaka M. Clinical study on aldolase isozyme--the development of the method of cancer diagnosis with muscle type aldolase. Hokkaido Igaku Zasshi 1979; 54:365-377

Asaka M, Nagase K, Shiraishi T, Miyazaki T. Diagnosis of
cancer by radioimmunoassay of muscle type aldolase. Gann
1980; 71:433-440

Asanami S. Studies on liver glucose-6-phosphate dehydrogenase and 6-phosphogluconate dehydrogenase of Erlich
ascites tumor-bearing mice. Shikwa Gakuho 1979; 79:
361-368

Ashall F, Bramwell ME, Harris H. A new marker for human
cancer cells. 1. The Ca antigen and the Ca1 antibody.
Lancet 1982; 8288:1-6

Atryzek V, Tamaoki T, Fausto N. Changes in polysomal
polyadenylated RNA and alpha-fetoprotein messenger RNA
during hepatocarcinogenesis. Cancer Res 1980; 40:
3713-3718

Aussel C, Lafaurie M, Stora C. Role physiologique de
l'alpha-faetoproteine (AFP). Effet d'injection d'AFP
purifee sur l'activite ovarienne du rat femelle adulte.
CR Acad Sci (D) Paris 1981; 292:553-556

Aussel C, Stora C, Lafaurie M, Krebs B, Ferrua B. Changes
in ovarian activity during hepatocarcinogenesis by N-2-
fluorenylacetamide: Role of alpha-fetoprotein. Steroids
1979; 34:631-642

Autio K, Turunen O, Eramaa E, Penttila O, Schroder J. Human
chronic lymphocytic leukaemia. Surface markers and activation of lymphocytes. Scand J Haematol 1979; 23:265-271

Ayeni RO, Tataryn DN, MacFarlane JK, Thomson DMP. A comput-
erized tube leukocyte adherence inhibition assay to detect
antitumor immunity in early human cancer: A review of two
years' experience. Surgery 1980; 87:380-389

Bagshawe KD, Searle F. Tumor markers. Essays Med Biochem
1977; 3:25-73

Baldwin RW, Robins RA. Interference with immunological
rejection of tumors. Br Med Bull 1976; 32:118-123

Baldwin RW, Robins RA. Circulating immune complexes in
cancer. In: Cancer Markers: Diagnostic and Developmental Significance. Sell S. ed. Clifton NJ: Humana
Press. 1980. pp. 507-531

Balinsky D. Enzymes and isozymes in cancer. In: Cancer
Markers: Diagnostic and Developmental Significance.
Sell S. ed. Clifton NJ: Humana Press. 1980.
pp. 191-224

Balis ME, Salser JS, Trotta PP, Wainfan E. Enzymes of
purine and pyrimidine metabolism as tumor markers. In:
Biological Markers of Neoplasia: Basic and Applied
Aspects. Ruddon RW. ed. New York: Elsevier North
Holland. 1978. pp. 517-534

Ballantyne B, Bright JE. Variations in mammalian renal
cortical beta-glucuronidase activity according to species,
strain and sex. Cell Mol Biol 1978; 23:369-378

Bara J, Paul-Gardais A, Loisillier F, Burtin P. Isolation
of a sulfated glycopeptidic antigen from human gastric
tumors: Its localization in normal and cancerous gastrointestinal tissues. Int J Cancer 1978; 21:133-139

Barthold SW. Relationship of colonic mucosal background
to neoplastic proliferative activity in dimethylhydrazine-
treated mice. Cancer Res 1981; 41:2616-2620

Bauer HW, Krause H. Variations in the level of the
pregnancy-associated α_2-glycoprotein in patients with
gynaecologic cancer. Eur J Cancer 1980; 16:1475-1481

Baylin SB, Mendelsohn G. Ectopic (inappropriate) hormone
production by tumors: Mechanisms involved and the biological and clinical implications. Endocr Rev 1980; 1:45-77

Beck PR, Belfield A, Spooner RJ. Serum enzymes in the diagnosis of hepatic metastatic carcinoma. Clin Chem 1978;
24:839

Becker U, Timpl R, Helle O, Porockop DJ. NH_4-terminal
extensions on skin collagen from sheep with a genetic
defect in conversion of procollagen to collagen.
Biochemistry 1976; 15:2853-2862

Beckley S, Chu TM, Wajsman Z, Mittelman A, Slack N,
Murphy GP. Modern concepts of acid and alkaline phosphatase measurement. Scand J Respir Dis Suppl 1980; 55:65-70

Bekesi JG, Tsang P, Holland JF. Specific role of T-lymphocytes in the ^{51}Cr-leukocyte adherence inhibition in the

diagnosis of cancer. Proc Am Assoc Cancer Res 1982;
23:260

Bell CE Jr, Seetharam S. A plasma membrane antigen highly
associated with oat-cell carcinoma of the lung and undetectable in normal adult tissue. Int J Cancer 1976;
18:605-611

Bell CE Jr, Seetharam S. Expression of endodermally derived
and neural crest-derived differentiation antigens by human
lung and colon tumors. Cancer 1979; 44:13-18

Belnap LP, Cleveland PH, Colmerauer ME, Barone RM, Pilch YH.
Immunogenicity of chemically induced murine colon cancers.
Cancer Res 1979; 39:1174-1179

Belville WD, Cox HD, Mahan DE, Stutzman RE, Bruce AW. Prostatic acid phosphatase by radioimmunoassay tumor marker in
bone marrow. J Urol 1979; 121:442-446

Bender JW. Serum phosphodiesterase I activity in breast
cancer patients. Med Pediatr Oncol 1979; 7:401-404

Bennett C, Cooke KB. Further characterization of a
melanoma-specific protein from human urine. Br J Cancer
1980; 41:734-744

Bernacki RJ, Kim U. Concomitant elevations in serum sialyltransferase activity and sialic acid content in rats with
metastasizing mammary tumors. Science 1977; 195:577-579

Betkerur V, Hliang V, Baumgartner G, Rao R, Albin RJ,
Guinan PD. Screening tests for the detection of bladder
cancer. Allergol Immunopathol 1980a; 8:169-176

Betkerur V, Hliang V, Baumgartner G, Rao R, Albin RJ,
Guinan PD. Screening tests for detection of bladder
cancer. Urology 1980b; 16:16-19

Bhattacharya M, Barlow JJ. Tumor markers for ovarian
cancer. Int Adv Surg Oncol 1979; 2:155-176

Bhattacharya M, Chatterjee SK, Barlow JJ. Uridine-5'-
diphosphate-galactose: Glycoprotein galactosyltransferase
activity in the ovarian cancer patient. Cancer Res 1976;
36:2096-2101

Bishop JM. Enemies within: The genesis of retrovirus
oncogenes. Cell 1981; 23:5-6

Bishop JM. Oncogenes. Sci Am 1982; 246:81-92

Black MM, Zachrau RE, Shore B, Leis HP Jr. Biological
   considerations of tumor-specific and virus-associated
   antigens of human breast cancers. Cancer Res 1976;
   36:769-774

Bloom SR, Polak JM, Pearse AG. Vasoactive intestinal
   peptide and watery-diarrhoea syndrome. Lancet 1973;
   819:14-16

Boelsterli U. Gamma-glutamyl transpeptidase (GGT)--an early
   marker for hepatocarcinogens in rats. Trends Pharmacol
   Sci 1979; 1:47-49

Boelsterli U, Zbinden G. Application of fine-needle aspiration biopsy for the diagnosis of dysplastic and neoplastic
   liver cell changes induced by N-nitrosomorpholine in rats.
   Arch Toxicol 1979; 42:225-238

Boettiger LE, Lindstedt S, von Schrreb T. Determination
   of lactic dehydrogenase in the urine as an aid to the
   diagnosis of cancer of the kidney. Acta Chir Scand 1966;
   132:356-361

Bohuon C, Assicot M. Polyamines as tumor markers. In:
   Cancer Related Antigens. Proc Eur Econ Commun Symp 1976;
   125-130

Bollum FJ. Terminal deoxynucleotidyl transferase as hematopoietic cell marker. Blood 1979; 54:1203-1215

Borek E. Transfer RNA and its by-products as tumor markers.
   In: Cancer Markers: Diagnostic and Developmental
   Significance. Sell S. ed. Clifton NJ: Humana Press.
   1980. pp. 445-462

Borek E, Kerr SJ. Atypical transfer RNAs and their origin
   in neoplastic cells. Adv Cancer Res 1972; 15:163-190

Borenfreund E, Bendich A. In vitro demonstration of Mallory
   body formation in liver cells from rats fed diethylnitrosamine. Lab Invest 1978; 38:295-303

Borenfreund E, Higgins P, Peterson E. Intermediate-sized
   filaments in cultured rat liver tumor cells with Mallory
   body-like cytoplasm abnormalities. J Nat Cancer Inst
   1980; 64:323-333

Bosl GJ, Lange PH, Nochomovitz LE, Goldmann A, Fraley EE, Rosai J, Johnson K, Kennedy BJ. Tumor markers in advanced nonseminomatous testicular cancer. Cancer 1981; 47: 572-576

Bosmann HB, Hall TC. Enzyme activity in invasive tumors of human breast and colon. Proc Nat Acad Sci USA 1974; 71: 1833-1837

Bosmann HB, Hilf R. Elevations in serum glycoprotein: N-Acetylneuraminic acid transferases in rats bearing mammary tumors. FEBS Lett 1974; 44:313

Bosmann HB, Spataru AC, Myers MW. Serum and host liver activities of glycosidases and sialytransferases in animals bearing transplantable tumors. Res Commun Chem Pathol Pharmacol 1975; 12:449-512

Bowman PW, Melvin SL, Aur RJA, Maner AM. A clinical perspective on cell markers in acute lymphocytic leukemia. Cancer Res 1981; 41:4794-4801

Boyd JN, Misslbeck N, Babish JG, Campbell TC, Stoeswand GS. Plasma alpha-fetoprotein elevation and mutagenicity of urine as early predictors of carcinogenicity in benzo(α)-pyrene fed rats. Drug Chem Toxicol 1981; 4:197-205

Boyd JN, Stoewsand GS, Misslbeck N, Campbell TC, Mason R, Lepp CA, Odstrchel G. Enhancement of plasma alpha-fetoprotein, as measured by sandwich-type radioimmunoassay, and induction of gamma-glutamyl transpeptidase-positive hepatic cell foci in rats fed benzo(a)pyrene. J Toxicol Environ Health 1981; 7:1025-1035

Bradstock KF, Janossy G, Hoffbrand AV, Ganeshagum K, Llewellin P, Prentice HG, Bollum FJ. Immunofluorescent and biochemical studies of terminal deoxynucleotidyl transferase in treated acute leukemia. Br J Haematol 1981; 47:121-131

Brattain MG, Green C, Kimball PM, Marks M, Khaled M. Isoenzymes of beta-hexosaminidase from normal rat colon and colonic carcinoma. Cancer Res 1979; 39:4083-4090

Braun JP, Rico AG, Benard P, Burgat-Sacaze V. Gamma-glutamyltransferase from human pathology to animal biology. Ann Biol Clin 1977; 35:433-447

Braunstein GD. Hormones: New potential for tumor markers. In: Diagnostic Medicine. June 1981. pp 1-7

Broder LE, Weintraub BD, Rosen SW, Cohen MH, Tejada F. Placental proteins and their subunits as tumor markers in prostatic carcinoma. Cancer 1977; 40:211-216

Brown CA. The cytochemical demonstration of beta-glucuronidase in colon neoplasms of rats exposed to azoxymethane. J Histochem Cytochem 1978; 26:22-27

Brown CE, Warren S, Chute RN, Ryan KJ, Todd RB. Hormonally induced tumors of the reproductive system of parabiosed male rats. Cancer Res 1979; 39:3971-3976

Brown PR, Krstulovic AM, Hartwick RA. Current state of the art in the HPLC analyses of free nucleotides, nucleosides, and bases in biological fluids. Adv Chromatogr 1980; 18:101-138

Brunner H, Schiller G. Significance of gamma-glutamyl-transpeptidase in the diagnosis of liver diseases. Fortschr Med 1977; 95:287-290

Bubenik J, Cochran AJ, Todd G, Malkovsky M, Jandlova T, Suhajova E, Boubelik M. A comparison of the macrophage electrophoretic mobility test and the leukocyte migration inhibition test in the detection of histocompatibility antigens on tumor cells. Neoplasma 1981; 28:185-193

Bubenikova D, Bubenik J, Holusa R, Svoboda V. Cell-surface adhesiveness of mouse leukemias. Neoplasma 1980; 27: 151-157

Bull RJ, Pereira MA. Development of a short-term testing matrix for estimating relative carcinogenic risk. J Am Coll Toxicol 1982; 1:1-15

Bumol TF, Ritzel EF, Douglas SD, Basch RS, Buxbaum JH, Faras AJ. Terminal deoxynucleotidyl transferase expression in a Thy-1 alloantigen variant lymphoma cell line. Immunology 1980; 41:799-806

Burrows S. Serum enzymes in the diagnosis of ovarian malignancy. Am J Obstet Gynecol 1980; 137:140-141

Busch H, Yeoman LC. eds. Tumor markers: In: Methods
in Cancer Research, Vol. 19. New York: Academic Press.
1982. 423 pp

Busch H, Yeoman LC. eds. Tumor markers. In: Methods
in Cancer Research, Vol. 20. New York: Academic Press.
1982. 400 pp

Butler WH, Hempsall V. Histochemical observations on
nodules induced in the mouse liver by phenobarbitone.
J Pathol 1978; 125:155-161

Butler WH, Hempsall V. Histochemical studies of hepatocellular carcinomas in the rat induced by aflatoxin.
J Pathol 1981; 134:157-170

Butler WH, Hempsall V, Stewart MG. Histochemical studies
on the early proliferative lesion induced in the rat liver
by aflatoxin. J Pathol 1981; 133:325-340

Cadeau BJ, Blackstein ME, Malkin A. Increased incidence of
placenta-like alkaline phosphatase activity in breast and
genitourinary cancer. Cancer Res 1974; 34:729-732

Cameron R, Lee G, Parker NB. Increased epoxide hydrase
activity following aflatoxin B$_1$, diethylnitrosamine (DEN),
2-acetylaminofluorene (2-AAF), safrole and azo dye administration, and in hyperplastic nodules and hepatomas
induced by DEN and 2-AAF. Proc Am Assoc Cancer Res 1979;
20:50

Cameron R, Sweeney GD, Jones K, Lee G, Farber EA. Relative
deficiency of cytochrome P-450 and aryl hydrocarbon
hydroxylase in hyperplastic nodules induced by 2-acetyl-
aminofluorene in rat liver. Cancer Res 1976; 36:3888-3893

Campanacci M, Bertoni F, Capanna R. Malignant degeneration
in fibrous dysplasia (presentation of 6 cases and review
of the literature). Ital J Orthop Traumatol 1979; 5:
373-381

Canellakis ES, Viceps-Madore D, Kyriakidis DA, Heller JS.
The regulation and function of ornithine decarboxylase and
of the polyamines. Curr Top Cell Regul 1979; 15:155-202

Carney DN, Marangos PJ, Ihde DC, Bunn PA Jr, Cohen MH,
Minna JD, Gazdar AF. Serum neuron-specific enolase:

A marker for disease extent and response to therapy of small-cell lung cancer. Lancet 1982; 8272:583-585

Carpentier NA, Fiere DM, Schuh D, Lange GT, Lainbert P. Circulating immune complexes and the prognosis of acute myeloid leukemia. New Engl J Med 1982; 307:1174-1180.

Castor CW, Cobel-Geard SR, Hossler PA, Kelch RP. Connective tissue activation. XXII. A platelet growth factor (connective tissue-activating peptide-III) in human growth hormone-deficient patients. J Clin Endocrinol Metab 1981; 52:128-132

Catalona WJ, Menon M. New screening and diagnostic tests for prostate cancer and immunologic assessment. Urology 1981; 17:61-65

Cater KC, Gandolfi AJ, Sipes JG. An evaluation of dimethyl-nitrosamine (DMN)-induced hepatocellular alterations in the newborn mouse model using histochemical and histoenzymatic markers. Toxicologist 1982; 1:99

Catovsky D, de Salvo Cardullo L, O'Brien M, Morilla R, Costello C, Galton D, Ganeshaguru D, Hoffbrand V. Cytochemical markers of differentiation in acute leukemia. Cancer Res 1981; 41:4824-4832

Cha CM, Mastrofrancesco B, Cha S, Randall HT. Electrophoretic patterns of alkaline phosphatase isoenzymes in human sera with abnormally high activity, and an unusual band observed in sera of patients with pancreatic cancer. Clin Chem 1975; 21:1067-1071

Chaimoff C, Wolloch Y, Eichhorn F, Dintsman M. Gamma-glutamyl transpeptidase as an aid in the diagnosis of liver metastases. Isr J Med Sci 1975; 11:781-784

Chan JYH, Becker FF. Decreased fidelity of DNA polymerase activity during N-2-fluorenylacetamide hepatocarcinogenesis. Proc Nat Acad Sci USA 1979; 76:814-818

Chang MLW, Schuster EM, Lee JA, Snodgrass C, Benton DA. Effect of diet, dietary regimens and strain differences on some enzyme activities in rat tissues. J Nutr 1968; 96:368-374

Charman HP, Rahman R, White MH, Kim N, Gilden RV. Radio-immunoassay for the major structural protein of Mason-

Pfizer monkey virus: Attempts to detect the presence of antigen or antibody in humans. Int J Cancer 1977; 19:498-504

Chatterjee SK, Bhattacharya M, Barlow JJ. Glycosyltransferase and glycosidase activities in ovarian cancer patients. Cancer Res 1979; 39:1943-1951

Chatterjee SK, Bhattacharya M, Barlow JJ. Evaluation of 5'-nucleotidase as an enzyme marker in ovarian carcinoma. Cancer 1981; 47:2648-2653

Chawla RK, Wadsworth AD, Rudman D. Relation of the urinary cancer-related glycoprotein EDC1 to plasma inter-alpha-trypsin inhibitor. J Immunol 1977; 121:1636-1639

Chheda GB. Purine and pyrimidine derivatives excreted in human urine. In: Handbook of Biochemistry, 2nd ed. Sober HA. ed. Cleveland OH: The Chemical Rubber Co. 1970. pp. G106-G113

Chien M-C, Tong MJ, Lo KJ, Lee JK, Millch DR, Vyas GN, Murphy BL. Hepatitis B viral markers in patients with primary hepatocellular carcinoma in Taiwan. J Nat Cancer Inst 1981; 66:475-479

Chio LF, Oon CJ. Changes in serum α_1-antitrypsin, α_1-acid glycoprotein and β_1-glycoprotein I in patients with malignant hepatocellular carcinoma. Cancer 1979; 43:596-604

Chiu JF, Pumo D, Gootnick D. Antigenic changes in nuclear chromatin in 1,2-dimethylhydrazine-induced colon carcinogenesis. Cancer 1980; 45:1193-1198

Chu TM. ed. Clinical and Biochemical Analysis: Biochemical Markers for Cancer. New York: Marcel Dekker, Inc. 1982. p. 375

Chu TM, Holyoke ED, Cedermark R, Evans J, Fisher D. A long-term follow-up of CEA in resective colorectal cancer. In: Oncodevelopmental Gene Expression. Fishman WH, Sell S. eds. New York: Academic Press. 1976. p. 427

Chu TM, Reynoso G, Hansen HJ. Demonstration of carcino-embryonic antigen in normal human plasma. Nature 1972; 238:152-153

Chu TM, Wang MC, Lee CL, Killian CS, Valenzuela LA, Wajsman Z, Slack N, Murphy GP. Enzyme markers for prostate cancer. In: Cancer Detect Prev 1980; Vol 2. New York: Elsevier. 680 pp.

Cimitan M, Busnardo B, Girelli ME, Casara D, Zanatta GP. Carcinoembryonic antigen in thyroid cancer. J Endocrinol Invest 1979; 2:241-244

Claflin AJ, McKinney EC, Fletcher MA. Immunological studies of prostate adenocarcinoma in an animal model. Prog Clin Biol Res 1980; 37:365-377

Clampitt RB. An investigation into the value of some clinical biochemical tests in the detection of minimal changes in liver morphology and function in the rat. Arch Toxicol Suppl 1978; 1:1-13

Clawson GA, Woo CH, Smuckler EA. Independent responses of nucleoside triphosphatase and protein kinase activities in nuclear envelope following thioacetamide treatment. Biochem Biophys Res Commun 1980; 95:1200-1204

Coakham HB, Kornblith PL, Quindlen EA, Pollock LA, Wood WC, Hartnett LC. Autologous humoral response to human gliomas and analysis of certain cell surface antigens: In vitro study with the use of microtoxicity and immune adherence assays. J Nat Cancer Inst 1980; 64:223-233

Coffey DS, Isaacs JT. Requirements for an idealized animal model of prostatic cancer. Prog Clin Biol Res 1980; 37:379-391

Coleman MS, Greenwood MF, Hutton JJ, Bollum FJ, Lampkin B, Holland P. Serial observations on terminal deoxynucleotidyl transferase activity and lymphoblast surface markers in acute lymphoblastic leukemia. Cancer Res 1976; 36:120-127

Constanza ME, Das S, Nathanson L, Rule A, Schwartz RS. Carcinoembryonic antigen: Report of a screening study. Cancer 1974; 33:583

Coombes RC. Calcitonin as a tumor marker: A review of interlaboratory determinations. Linand Rev 1980; 80:53-55

Coombes RC, Ellison MI, Neville AM. Biochemical markers in bronchogenic carcinoma. Br J Dis Chest 1978; 72:263-287

Coombes RC, Powles TJ, Gazet JC, Nash AG, Ford HT, McKinna A, Neville AM. Assessment of biochemical tests to screen for metastasis in patients with breast cancer. Lancet 1980; 1:296-297

Coombes RC, Powles TJ, Gazet JC, Ford HT, McKinna A, Abbott M, Gehrke CW, Keyser JW, Mitchell PEG, Patel S, Stimson WH, Worwood M, Jones M, Neville AM. Screening for metastases in breast cancer: An assessment of biochemical and physical methods. Cancer 1981; 48:310-315

Coombes RC, Powles TJ, Gazet JC, Ford HT, Sloane JP, Laurence DJR, Neville AM. Biochemical markers in human breast cancer. Lancet 1977; 1:132-134

Coombes RC, Powles TJ, Neville AM. Evaluation of biochemical markers in breast cancer. Proc R Soc Med 1977; 70:843-845

Cooper EH, Plesner T. Beta-2-microglobulin review: Its relevance in clinical oncology. Med Pediatr Oncol 1980; 8:323-334

Cooper GM, Okenquist S, Silverman L. Transforming activity of DNA of chemically transformed and normal cells. Nature 1980; 284:418-421

Cooper IA, Wray GR, Murphy TL. Urinary excretory patterns of tRNA degradation products: A marker of Hodgkin's cell metabolism? Eur J Cancer 1977; 13:1309-1312

Cornish HH. Problems posed by observations of serum enzyme changes in toxicology. CRC Crit Rev Toxicol 1971; 1:1-32

Costa M, Nye JS, Suderman FW Jr, Allpass PR, Gondos B. Induction of sarcomas in nude mice by implantation of Syrian hamster fetal cells exposed in vitro to nickel subsulfide. Cancer Res 1979; 39:3591-3597

Covington EE, D'Angio GJ, Helson L, Romano RW. Seleno-methionine 75 as a scanning agent for neuroblastoma. Clin Bull 1974; 4:147-150

Cowen DM, Searle F, Ward AM, Benson EA, Smiddy FG, Eaves G, Cooper EH. Multivariate biochemical indicators in breast cancer: An evaluation of their potential in routine practice. Eur J Cancer 1978; 14:885-893

Crampton RF, Gray TJB, Grasso P, Parke DV. Long-term studies on chemically induced liver enlargement in the rat. I. Sustained induction of microsomal enzymes with absence of liver damage on feeding phenobarbitone or butylated hydroxytoluene. Toxicology 1977a; 7:289-306

Crampton RF, Gray TJB, Grasso P, Parke DV. Long-term studies on chemically induced liver enlargement in the rat. II. Transient induction of microsomal enzymes leading to liver damage and nodular hyperplasia produced by safrole and Ponceau MX. Toxicology 1977b; 7:307-326

Culling CFA. Handbook of Histopathological and Histochemical Techniques, 3rd ed. London: Butterworth. 1974

Culvenor JG, Harris AW, Mandel TE, Whitelaw A, Ferber E. Alkaline phosphatase in hematopoietic tumor cell lines of the mouse: High activity in cells of the B lymphoid lineage. J Immunol 1981; 126:1974-1977

Cummins RR, Balinsky O. Activities of some enzymes of pyrimidine and DNA synthesis in a rat transplantable hepatoma and human primary hepatomas, in cell lines derived from these tissues, and in human fetal liver. Cancer Res 1980; 40:1235-1239

Curtin NJ, Snell K. Changes in developmental-specific enzyme activities during experimental hepatocarcinogenesis in the rat in vivo. Biochem Soc Trans 1980; 8:94

Dacha U, Sensini A, Giacchi R, Canestrari F, Palma F, Dacha M, Faggioni A. Modification of the hetokinase activity in the red blood cells of subjects with differentiated adenocarcinoma. Tumori 1980; 66:43-49

Damle SR, Shetty PA, Jussawalla DJ, Bhide SV, Baxi AJ. Occurrence of heat-labile Regan type of alkaline phosphatase in hematopoietic tumors. Int J Cancer 1979; 24: 398-401

Dao TL, Ip C, Patel J. Serum sialyltransferase and 5'-nucleotidase as reliable biomarkers in women with breast cancer. J Nat Cancer Inst 1980; 65:529-534

Davey FR, Huntington SJ, MacCallum J, MacMath JM. Cytochemical reactions of normal and neoplastic lymphocytes. J Clin Pathol 1977; 30:653-660

Davis GE, Gehrke CW, Kuo KC, Agris PF. Major and modified
nucleosides in tRNA hydrolysates by high performance
liquid chromatography. J Chromatogr 1979; 173:281-289

Davis TE, Kahan L, Tormey DC, Larson FC, Anderson SA,
Crowley JJ, Carey RN. Clinical studies of a fast
homoarginine-sensitive alkaline phosphatase in patients
with cancer. Cancer Res 1981; 41:1110-1113

De Gerlache J, Lans M, Taper H, Roberfroid M. Separate
isolation of cells from nodules and surrounding parenchyma
of the same precancerous rat liver: Biochemical and cytochemical characterization. Toxicology 1980; 18:225-232

DeLeo AB, Jay G, Appella E, DuBois GC, Law LW, Old LJ. Cell
surface antigens of chemically induced sarcomas of inbred
mice. Transplant Proc 1980; 12:65-69

De Luca M, Hall N, Rice R, Kaplan NO. Creatine kinase isozymes in human tumors. Biochem Biophys Res Commun 1981;
99:189-195

Denk H, Franke WW, Kerjaschki D, Eckerstorfer R. Mallory
bodies in experimental animals and man. Int Rev Exp
Pathol 1979; 20:77-121

Dent JG. Hepatic epoxide hydratase: A possible biochemical marker for hepatocarcinogens. Toxicol Lett 1980;
61 Spec:115

Dent PB, McCulloch PB. Detection of recurrent metastasis
using tumor associated serum markers. Eur J Cancer 1980;
16:963

Dermer GB, Silverman LM, Gendler SJ, Tokes ZA. Incidence
of a split α_2-glycoprotein band in the electrophoretic
pattern for serum of adenocarcinoma patients. Clin Chem
1980; 26:392-395

Desser H, Lutz D, Krieger O, Stierer M. Rapid detection
of polyamines in the sera of patients with colorectal
carcinoma by liquid ion-exhange chromatography. Oncology
1980b; 37:376-380

Desser H, Niebauer GW, Gebhart W. Polyamine and histamine
contents in the blood of pigmented, depigmented and melanoma bearing Lipizzaner horses. Zentralbl Veterinaermed A
1980a; 27:45-53

De The G, Lenoir G. Comparative diagnosis of Epstein-Barr
    virus related diseases: Infectious mononucleosis,
    Burkitt's lymphoma, and nasopharyngeal carcinoma. In:
    Comparative Diagnosis of Viral Diseases, Vol. 1. Human
    and Related Viruses, Part A. Kurstak E, Kurstak C.
    eds. London: Academic Press. 1978. pp. 195-240

DeYoung NJ, Ashman LK, Ludbrook J, Marshall VR. A
    comparison of three blood tests for cancer. Surg Gynecol
    Obstet 1980; 150:12-16

Dobryszycka W, Warwas M, Gerber J, Vjec M. Serum enzymes
    in ovarian carcinoma. Neoplasma 1979; 26:737-743

Dodson M, Menon M. Consideration and implications of
    tumor antigenic expression. Surg Gynecol Obstet 1979;
    149:770-779

Dolbeare F, Vanderlaan M, Phares W. Alkaline phosphatase
    and acid arylamidase marker enzymes for normal and trans-
    formed WE-38 cells. J Histochem Cytochem 1980; 28:419-426

Doos WG, Saravis CA, Pusztazeri G, Burke B, Oh SK,
    Zamcheck N, Gottlieb LS. Tissue localization of zinc
    glycinate marker and carcinoembryonic antigen by immuno-
    fluorescence. II. Immunofluorescence microscopy. J Nat
    Cancer Inst 1978; 60:1375-1382

Dorfman LE, Amador E, Wacker WEC. Urinary lactic dehydroge-
    nase activity. II. Elevated activities for the diagnosis
    of carcinomas of the kidney and the bladder. Biochem Clin
    1963a; 2:44-55

Dorfman LE, Amador E, Wacker WEC. Urinary lactic dehydroge-
    nase activity. III. An analytical validation of the assay
    method. J Am Med Assoc 1963b; 184:1-6

Drago JR, Goldman LB, Maurer RE. Histology, histochemistry,
    and acid phosphatase of Noble (Nb) rat prostate adenocar-
    cinoma and treatment of androgen-dependent Nb rat prostate
    adenocarcinoma. J Nat Cancer Inst 1980; 64:931-937

Drake WP, Kopyta LP, Levy CC, Mardiney MR Jr. Alterations
    in ribonuclease activities in the plasma, spleen, and
    thymus of tumor-bearing mice. Cancer Res 1975; 35:322-324

Du JT, Sandoz JP, Tseng MT, Tamburro CH. Biochemical
    alterations in livers of rats exposed to vinyl chloride.
    J Toxicol Environ Health 1979; 5:1119-1132

Dunzendorfer U, Schumann W, Drahovsky D, Ohlenschlager G. Glycopeptides (FSH, LH, TSH, prolactin) and glycoproteins in patients with genitourinary cancer. Oncology 1981; 38:110–115

Durham JP, Gillies D, Baxter A, Lopez-Solis RO. The application of a simple, sensitive disc assay for sialyl-transferase activity to particulate and soluble enzyme preparations and its use in measuring enzymatic activity in human plasma samples. Clin Chim Acta 1979; 95:425–432

Dutu R, Nedelea M, Veluda G, Berculet V. Cytoenzymatic investigations on carcinomas of the cervix uteri. Acta Cytol 1980; 24:160–166

Ehrmeyer SL, Joiner BL, Kahan L, Larson FC, Metzenberg RL. A cancer-associated fast, homoarginine-sensitive electrophoretic form of serum alkaline phosphatase. Cancer Res 1978; 38:599–601

Elder MG, Wood EJ, Said J. A modification of the serum glucose-6-phosphatase assay. Clin Chim Acta 1972; 38: 211–215

Ellins PH, Van der Weyden MB, Medley G. Thymidine kinase isoenzymes in human malignant melanoma. Cancer Res 1981; 41:691–695

Enomoto K, Ying TS, Griffin MJ, Farber E. Immunohistochemical study of epoxide hydrolase during experimental liver carcinogenesis. Cancer Res 1981; 41:3281–3287

Enzyme Nomenclature. New York: Academic Press. 1978

Essigmann EM, Newberne PM. Enzymatic alterations in mouse hepatic nodules induced by a chlorinated hydrocarbon pesticide. Cancer Res 1981; 41:2823–2831

Evans AW, Johnson NW, Butcher RG. A quantitative cytochemical study of three oxidative enzymes during experimental oral carcinogenesis in the hamster. Br J Oral Surg 1980a; 18:3–6

Evans IM, Hilf R, Murphy M, Bosmann HB. Correlation of serum, tumor, and liver serum glycoprotein: N-Acetyl-neuraminic acid transferase activity with growth of the R32 30AC mammary tumor in rats and relationship of the serum activity to tumor burden. Cancer Res 1980b; 40: 3103–3111

Evstigneeff T, Clot P, Delacoux E. Gamma-glutamyltranspeptidase and hepatic diseases. Nouv Presse Med 1973; 2:1-5

Farber E. The sequential analysis of liver cancer induction. Biochim Biophys Acta 1980; 605:149-166

Farber E. Chemical carcinogenesis. New Engl J Med 1981;
305:1379-1389

Farber E. Chemical carcinogenesis: A biological perspective. Am J Pathol 1982; 106:271-296

Farber E, Cameron R. The sequential analysis of cancer
development. Adv Cancer Res 1980; 31:125-126

Farnsworth WE, Gonder MJ, Cartagena R, Steinbach JJ.
Comparative performance of three radioimmunoassays for
prostatic acid phosphatase. Urology 1980; 16:165-167

Farrell RJ. Biochemical markers in gynaecological cancer.
Ir Med J 1980; 73:285-286

Fenoglio CM. Antigens, enzymes and hormones. Diagn Gynecol
Obstet 1980; 2:33-42

Feron VJ, Kruysse A. Effects of exposure to acrolein vapor
in hamsters simultaneously treated with benzo(a)pyrene or
diethylnitrosamine. J Toxicol Environ Health 1977; 3:
379-394

Fiala S, Fiala AE, Keller RW, Fiala ES. Gamma glutamyl
transpeptidase in colon cancer induced by 1,2-dimethyl-
hydrazine. Arch Geschwulstforsch 1977; 47:117-122

Fiala S, Fiala ES. Activation by chemical carcinogens of
γ-glutamyl transpeptidase in rat and mouse liver. J Nat
Cancer Inst 1973; 51:151-158

Fiala S, Mohindru A, Kettering WG, Fiala AE, Morris HP.
Glutathione and gamma-glutamyl-transferase in rat liver
during chemical carcinogenesis. J Nat Cancer Inst 1976;
57:591-598

Fiala S, Reuber MD. High glutathionase in rat liver during
carcinogenesis. Gann 1970; 61:275-278

Fink K, Adams WS. Urinary purines and pyrimidines in normal
and leukemic subjects. Arch Biochem Biophys 1968; 126:
27-33

Fischer DR, Gevers W. Altered distribution of acid phosphatase in neoplastic prostatic cells. Urol Res 1980;
8:15-22

Fischer W, Grund E. The influence of 2-acetylaminofluorene
on the dietary induction of pentose phosphate pathway
enzymes. Arch Geschwulstforsch 1979; 49:381-385

Fishman L, Miyayama H, Driscoll SG, Fishman WH. Developmental phase-specific alkaline phosphatase isoenzymes of
human placenta and their occurrence in human cancer.
Cancer Res 1976; 36:2268-2273

Fishman WH. Perspectives on alkaline phosphatase isoenzymes. Am J Med 1974; 56:617-650

Fishman WH. Oncodevelopmental enzymes. In: The Clinical
Biochemistry of Cancer. Fleisher M. ed. Washington DC:
The American Association for Clinical Chemistry. 1979.
pp. 132-154

Fishman WH, Raam S, Stolbach LL. Markers for ovarian
cancer: Regan isoenzyme and other glycoproteins. Semin
Oncol 1975; 2:211-216

Foss ANG, Klepp O, Barth E, Aakvaag A, Kaalhus O.
Endocrinological studies in patients with metastatic
malignant testicular germ cell tumors. Int J Androl 1980;
3:487-501

Fritschle HA, Tashima CK, Collinsworth WL, Geifer A,
van Dort J. A direct competitive binding radioimmunoassay
for carcinoembryonic antigen. J Immunol Methods 1980;
35:115-128

Fu SM, Winchester RJ, Kunkel HG. Occurrence of surface IgM,
IgD, and free light chains on human lymphocytes. J Exp
Med 1974; 139:451-456

Fujisawa K, Kurihara N, Nishikawa H, Kimura A, Kojima M.
Carcinoembryonic character of gamma-glutamyltranspeptidase
in primary hepatocellular carcinoma. Gastroenterol Jpn
1976; 11:380-386

Fujisawa T, Waldman SR, Yonemoto RH. Leukocyte adherence
inhibition by soluble tumor antigens in breast cancer
patients. Cancer 1977; 39:506-513

Fujita D, Nagatsu T, Maruta K, Ito M, Senba H, Mike K. Urinary putrescine, spermidine, and spermine in human blood and solid cancers and in an experimental gastric tumor of rats. Cancer Res 1976; 36:1320-1324

Fujita K, Nagatsu T, Shinpo D, Maruta K, Takahashi H, Sekiya A. Increase of urinary putrescine in 3,4-benzopyrene carcinogenesis and its inhibition by putrescine. Cancer Res 1978; 38:3509-3511

Fuks A, Shuster J, Gold P. Theoretical and practical considerations of the utility of the radioimmunoassay for carcinoembryonic antigen (CEA) in clinical medicine. In: Cancer Markers: Diagnostic and Developmental Significance. Sell S. ed. Clifton NJ: Humana Press. 1980. pp. 315-327

Fukushima S, Shibata M, Hibino T, Yoshimura T, Hirose M, Ito N. Intrahepatic bile duct proliferation induced by 4,4'-diaminodiphenylmethane in rats. Toxicol Appl Pharmacol 1979; 48:145-155

Fulton DS, Levin VA, Lubich WP, Wilson CB, Marton LJ. Cerebrospinal fluid polyamines in patients with glioblastoma multiforme and anaplastic astrocytoma. Cancer Res 1980; 40:3293-3296

Gabbiani G, Trenchev P, Holbrow EJ. Increase in contractile proteins in human cancer cells. Lancet 1975; 2:796-797

Ganzinger U. Klinische Andwenbarkeit der Serum-Sialyltransferase-Bestimmung als Mass maligne transformierter Zelloberflächenstrukturen. Wien Klin Wochenschr 1977; 89:594-597

Ganzinger U, Deutsch E. Serum sialyltransferase levels as parameter in the diagnosis and follow-up of gastrointestinal tumors. Cancer Res 1980; 40:1300-1304

Gehrke CW, Kuo KC, Waalkes TP, Borek E. Urinary nucleosides as markers for diagnosis and the monitoring of therapy. In: Biological Markers of Neoplasia: Basic and Applied Aspects. Ruddon RW. ed. New York: Elsevier North Holland. 1978. pp. 559-567

Gerber MA, Garfinkel E, Hirschman SZ, Thung SN, Panagiotatos T. Immune and enzyme histochemical studies of a human hepatocellular carcinoma cell line producing hepatitis B surface antigen. J Immunol 1981: 126:1085-1089

Gerber MA, Thung SN. Enzyme patterns in human hepatocellular carcinoma. Am J Pathol 1980; 98:395-400

Ghanta VK, Hiramoto RN, Weiss A, Caudill L. Monitoring of murine osteosarcoma by serial alkaline phosphatase determination. J Nat Cancer Inst 1976; 57:837-839

Ghanta VK, Soong SJ, Hurst DC, Hiramoto RN. Osteosarcoma associated alkaline phosphatase and in vivo growth and development. Proc Soc Exp Biol Med 1980; 164:229-233

Gielen JE, Goujon F, Sele J, Van Cantfort J. Organ specificity of induction of activating and inactivating enzymes by cigarette smoke and cigarette smoke condensate. Arch Toxicol 1979; 41:239-251

Giler S, Kupfer B, Urca I, Moroz C. Immunodiagnostic test for the early detection of carcinoma of the breast. Surg Gynecol Obstet 1979; 149:655-657

Giler S, Moroz C. The significance of ferritin in malignant diseases. Biomedicine 1978; 28:203-206

Gilliland BC, Mannik M. Immune Complex Diseases. In: Harrison's Principles of Internal Medicine, 8th ed. Thorn GW et al. eds. New York: McGraw-Hill. 1977. pp. 409-413

Gold DV. Immunoperoxidase localization of colonic mucoprotein antigen in neoplastic disease. Cancer Res 1981; 41:767-772

Gold P, Freedman SO. Specific carcinoembryonic antigens of the human digestive system. J Exp Med 1965; 122:467-481

Goldberg DM, Martin JV. Role of gamma-glutamyl transpeptidase activity in the diagnosis of hepatobiliary disease. Digestion 1975; 12:232-246

Goldberg EM, Hansen H. GW-39, a tumor-animal model for carcinoembryonic antigen (CEA). Proc Am Assoc Cancer Res 1972; 13:80

Goldfarb S, Pugh TD. Enzyme histochemical phenotypes in primary hepatocellular carcinomas. Cancer Res 1981; 41:2092-2095

Goldfarb S, Pugh TD. The origin and significance of hyperplastic hepatocellular islands and nodules in hepatic carcinogenesis. J Am Coll Toxicol 1982; 1:119-144

Goldfarb S, Pugh TD, Cripps DJ. Increased alkaline phosphatase activity--a positive histochemical marker for griseofulvin-induced mouse hepatocellular nodules. J Nat Cancer Inst 1980; 64:1427-1433

Goldrosen MH, Dasmahapatra K, Jenkins D, Howell JH, Arbuck SG, Moore MC, Douglass HO Jr. Microplate leukocyte adherence inhibition (LAI) assay in pancreatic cancer. Cancer 1981; 47:1614-1619

Goldrosen MH, Russo AJ, Howell JH, Leveson SH, Holyoke ED. Cellular and humoral factors involved in the mechanism of the micro-leukocyte adherence inhibition reaction. Cancer Res 1979; 39:587-592

Goldrosen MH, Russo AJ, Howell JH, Leveson SH, Moore MC, Holyoke ED, Douglass MO Jr. Evaluation of micro-leukocyte adherence inhibition as an immunodiagnostic test for pancreatic cancer. Cancer Res 1979; 39:633-637

Gorsky Y, Sulitzeanu DA. Radioactive antibody binding-inhibition assay for the detection of cell-membrane related antigens in body fluids. J Immunol Methods 1975; 6:291-300

Goyette M, Petropoulos CJ, Shank PR, Fausto N. Expression of a cellular oncogene during liver regeneration. Science 1983; 219:510-512

Graichen ME, Dent JG. 2-Acetylaminofluorene (AAF) dependent increases in epoxide hydrolase: Species, strain and sex differences. Toxicologist 1982; 2:101

Gravela E, Feo F, Canuto RA, Garcea R, Gabriel C. Functional and structural alterations in liver ergastoplasmic membranes during DL-ethionine hepatocarcinogenesis. Cancer Res 1975; 35:3041-3047

Grayhack JT, Lee C, Kolbusz W, Oliver L. Detection of carcinoma of the prostate utilizing biochemical observations. Cancer 1980; 45:1896-1901

Greaves MF, Brown G, Rapson NT, Lister TA. Antisera to acute lymphoblastic leukemia cells. Clin Immunol Immunopathol 1975; 4:67-84

Greene FE, Jernstrom B. Epoxide hydratase and glutathione
    S-transferase activities in human lungs. Cancer Lett
    1980; 8:235-239

Greengard O. Detection of extrahepatic cancer by altera-
    tions in hepatic functions. Biochem Pharmacol 1979;
    28:2569-2572

Greiner JW, Malan-Shibley LB, Janss DH. Detection of aryl
    hydrocarbon hydroxylase activity in normal and neoplastic
    human breast epithelium. Life Sci 1980; 26:313-319

Grice HC. The changing role of pathology in modern safety
    evaluation. CRC Crit Rev Toxicol 1972; 1:119-152

Griffin MJ. Epoxide hydrolase and hepatocarcinogenesis.
    TIPS Rev 1981; 2:257-258

Griffing G, Vaitukaitis JL. Hormone-secreting tumors.
    In: Cancer Markers: Diagnostic and Developmental
    Significance. Sell S. ed. Clifton NJ: Humana Press.
    1980. pp. 169-190

Gropp C, Havemann K. Significance of tumor markers in the
    diagnosis and treatment of bronchial carcinoma. Onkologie
    1980; 3:133-138

Gropp C, Havemann K, Scherfe T, Ax W. Incidence of circula-
    ting immune complexes in patients with lung cancer and
    their effect on antibody-dependent cytotoxicity. Oncology
    1980; 37:71-76

Gropp C, Havemann K, Scheuer A. The use of carcinoembryonic
    antigen and peptide hormones to stage and monitor patients
    with lung cancer. Int J Radiat Oncol Biol Phys 1980; 6:
    1047-1053

Guy K, DiMario U, Irvine WJ, Hunter AM, Hadley A,
    Horne NW. Circulating immune complexes and autoantibodies
    in lung cancer. Br J Cancer 1981; 43:276-283

Haagensen DE Jr, Kister SJ, Panik J, Giannola J, Hansen HJ,
    Wells SA Jr. Comparative evaluation of carcinoembryonic
    antigen and gross cystic disease fluid protein as plasma
    markers for breast carcinoma. Cancer 1978; 42:1646-1652

Habeshaw JA, Catley PF, Stansfield AG, Ganeshaguru K,
    Hoffbrand AV. Terminal deoxynucleotidyl transferase
    activity in lymphoma. Br J Cancer 1979; 39:566-569

Hadley NA, Sindelar WF. Antifetal and tumor-specific reactivity in human osteosarcoma. Surg Forum 1979; 30:122-124

Hagen C, Lindholm J, Wuenson E, Riishede J, Hummer L, Jacobsen HH. Relationship between plasma prolactin concentration and pituitary function in patients with a pituitary adenoma. Clin Endocrinol 1979; 11:671-679

Hagerstrand I. Enzyme histochemistry of the liver in extrahepatic biliary obstruction. Acta Pathol Microbiol Scand 1973; 81:737-750

Haije WG, Meerwaldt JH, Talerman A, Kuipers TJ, Baggerman L, Teeuw AH, van der Pompe WB, van Driel J. The value of a sensitive assay of carcino-placental alkaline phosphatase (CPAP) in the follow-up of gynecological cancers. Int J Cancer 1979; 24:288-293

Haines HG, McCoy JP, Hofheinz DE, Ng ABP, Nordqvist SRB, Leif RC. Cervical carcinoma antigens in the diagnosis of human squamous cell carcinoma of the cervix. J Nat Cancer Inst 1981; 66:465-474

Hakkinen IP, Heinonen R, Inberg MV, Jarvi OH, Vaajalahti P, Viikari S. Clinicopathological study of gastric cancers and precancerous states detected by fetal sulfoglycoprotein antigen screening. Cancer Res 1980; 40:4308-4312

Hakomori S, Wang SM, Young WW Jr. Isoantigenic expression of Forssman glycolipid in human gastric and colonic mucosa: Its possible identity with "A-like antigen" in human cancer. Proc Nat Acad Sci USA 1977; 74:3023-3027

Hall RH. The Modified Nucleosides in Nucleic Acids. New York: Columbia University Press. 1971

Halliday WJ, Maluish AE, Stephenson PM, Davis NC. An evaluation of leukocyte adherence inhibition in the immunodiagnosis of colorectal cancer. Cancer Res 1977; 37:1962-1971

Halliday WJ, Miller S. Leukocyte adherence inhibition: A simple test for cell-mediated tumor immunity and serum blocking factors. Int J Cancer 1972; 9:477-483

Hammond KS, Papermaster DS. Fluorometric assay of sialic acid in the picomole range: A modification of the thiobarbituric acid assay. Anal Biochem 1976; 74:292-297

Hancock RC, Forrester PI, Lorscheider FL. Ethionine induced activation of embryonic genes. In: Oncodevelopmental Gene Expression. Fishman WH, Sell S. eds. New York: Academic Press. 1975. pp. 251-253

Hansen M, Hansen HH, Hirsch FR, Arends J, Christensen JD, Christensen JM, Hummer L, Kuhl C. Hormonal polypeptides and amine metabolites in small cell carcinoma of the lung, with special reference to stage and subtypes. Cancer 1980; 45:1432-1437

Harada F, Kuchino Y, Kawachi T, Nishimura S. Excretion of cytidine, deoxycytidine and pseudourine in urine of rats bearing Morris hepatoma 7794A. Proceedings Japanese Cancer Association, 32nd Annual Meeting. 1973. p. 108

Harada M, Okabe K, Shibata K, Masuda H, Miyata K, Enomoto M. Histochemical demonstration of increased activity of γ-glutamyl transpeptidase in rat liver during hepatocarcino-genesis. Acta Histochem Cytochem 1976; 9:168-179

Harper HA. Review of Physiological Chemistry, 12th ed. Los Altos CA: Lange Medical Publications. 1969. p. 349

Harris H, Bramwell ME, McGee JO. Ca antigen is not Thomsen-Friedenreich antigen [Letter]. Lancet (England) 1982; 8304:925-926

Harris PA, Stephens RW, Ghosh P, Taylor TK. Endo- and exoglycosidases in an experimental rat osteosarcoma. Aust J Exp Biol Med Sci 1977; 55:363-370

Haselager EM, Vreeken J. Clinical significance of circulating fibrin monomers. J Clin Pathol 1981; 34:468-472

Hautmann R. Diagnosis of renal disorders: Comparison of urinary enzyme patterns with corresponding tissue patterns. Curr Probl Clin Biochem 1979; 9:58-70

Hayes JR, Campbell TC. Nutrition as a modifier of chemical carcinogenesis. In: Carcinogenesis: Modifiers of Chemical Carcinogenesis, Vol. 5. Slaga TJ. ed. New York: Raven Press. 1980. pp. 207-241

Heaney JA, Lin JC, Daly JJ, Prout GR Jr. Immunological detection of metastases from prostatic adenocarcinoma. J Surg Oncol 1981; 14:83-88

Heinle H, Wendel A, Schmidt U. The activities of the key enzymes of the γ-glutamyl cycle in microdissected segments of the rat nephron. FEBS Lett 1977; 77:220

Henderson M, Kessel D. Alterations in plasma sialyltransferase levels in patients with neoplastic disease. Cancer 1977; 39:1129-1134

Henry RC, Cannon DC, Winkel JW. Clinical Chemistry Principles and Techniques, 2nd ed. Hagerstown MD: Harper and Row. 1974. pp. 608-615

Herberman RB. ed. Natural Cell-Mediated Immunity Against Tumors. New York: Academic Press. 1980. 1321 pp

Herzfeld A, Greengard O. Enzyme activities in human fetal and neoplastic tissues. Cancer 1980; 46:2047-2054

Herzfeld A, Greengard O, McDermott WV. Enzyme pathology of the liver in patients with and without nonhepatic cancer. Cancer 1980; 45:2383-2388

Herzfeld A, Raper SM. Amino acid metabolizing enzymes in rat submaxillary gland, normal or neoplastic, and in pancreas. Enzyme 1976; 21:471-480

Hetland O, Andersson TR, Gerner T. The heterogeneity of the serum activity of gamma-glutamyl transpeptidase in hepatobiliary diseases as studied by agarose gel electrophoresis. Clin Chim Acta 1975; 62:425-431

Hildebrand J. Early diagnosis of brain metastases in an unselected population of cancerous patients. Eur J Cancer 1973; 9:621-626

Hirai H. Alpha fetoprotein. In: Biochemical Markers for Cancer: Clinical and Biochemical Analysis, Vol. 11. Chu TM. ed. New York: Marcel Dekker, Inc. 1982. pp. 25-49

Hiramoto R, Ghanta V, Soong S, Hurst D. An experimental approach to relate a tumor-associated enzyme marker to tumor cell numbers. Cancer Res 1977; 37:365-368

Hirota N, Williams GM. The sensitivity and heterogeneity of histochemical markers for altered foci involved in liver carcinogenesis. Am J Pathol 1979; 95:317-328

Ho AD, Hunstein W, Dorken B, Pfreundschuh M, Kaufmann M, Kruger C. Leukocyte alkaline phosphatase in malignancies. Blut 1979; 39:141-145

Höffken K, Meredith ID, Robins RA, Baldwin RW, Davies CJ, Blamey RW. Circulating immune complexes in patients with breast cancer. Br Med J 1977; 2:218-220

Höffken K, Price MR, McLaughlin PJ, Moore VE, Baldwin RW. Circulating immune complexes in rats bearing chemically induced tumours. I. Sequential determination during the growth of tumours at various body sites. Int J Cancer 1978a; 21:496-504

Höffken K, Price MR, Moore VE, Baldwin RW. Circulating immune complexes in rats bearing chemically induced tumours. II. Characterization of sera from different stages of tumour growth. Int J Cancer 1978b; 22:576-582

Hoffmann W, Werner W, Steiner R, Kaufmann R. Cell electrophoresis for diagnostic purposes. I. Diagnostic value of the electrophoretic mobility test (EMT) for the detection of gynaecological malignancies. Br J Cancer 1981a; 43: 588-597

Hoffmann W, Kaufmann R, Steiner R, Werner W. Cell electrophoresis for diagnostic purposes. II. Critical evaluation of conventional cytopherometry. Br J Cancer 1981b; 43: 598-609

Hogan-Ryan A, Fennely JJ, Jones M, Cantwell B, Duffy MJ. Serum sialic acid and CEA concentrations in human breast cancer. Br J Cancer 1980; 41:587-592

Hollinshead AC. Analysis of soluble melanoma cell membrane antigens in metastatic cells of various organs and further studies of antigens present in primary melanoma. Cancer 1975; 35:1282-1288

Hollinshead AC, Chuang CY. Evaluation of the relationship of prealbumin components in sera of patients with cancer. Nat Cancer Inst Monogr 1978; 49:187-192

Hollinshead AC, Jaffurs WR, Alpert LK, Harris JE, Herberman RB. Isolation and identification of soluble skin-reactive membrane antigens of malignant and normal human breast cells. Cancer Res 1974; 34:2961-2968

Holyoke ED, Douglass HO Jr, Goldrosen MH, Chu TM. Tumor markers in pancreatic cancer. Semin Oncol 1979; 6:347-356

Homma H. Pro-ACTH as one of the biochemical markers in bronchogenic carcinoma. Igaku no Ayumi 1980; 113:945-952

Horne CH, Reid IN, Milne GD. Prognostic significance of inappropriate production of pregnancy proteins by breast cancers. Lancet 1976; 2:279-282

Horne CHW, Bremner RD. Pregnancy proteins as tumor markers. In: Cancer Markers: Diagnostic and Developmental Significance. Sell S. ed. Clifton NJ: Humana Press. 1980. pp. 225-247

Huber H, Douglas SD, Fudenberg HH. The IgG receptor: An immunological marker for the characterization of mono-nuclear cells. Immunology 1969; 17:7-21

Huguier M, Lacaine F. Hepatic metastases in gastrointes-tinal cancer: Diagnostic value of biochemical investiga-tions. Arch Surg 1981; 116:399-401

Hutchinson DR, Halliwell RP, Lockhart JD, Parke DV. Glycyl-prolyl-p-nitroanilidase in hepatobiliary disease. Clin Chim Acta 1981; 109:83-89

Hutter JJ Jr, Glasser L, Meyskens FL. Advances in the classification of acute leukemia in children. Ariz Med 1978; 35:345-348

IARC. International Agency for Research on Cancer. Monographs on the Evaluation of the Carcinogenic Risk of Chemicals to Humans. Chemicals, Industrial Processes and Industries Associated with Cancer in Humans, Suppl 4. 1982

Ideo G, Morganti A, Dioguardi N. γ-Glutamyl transpeptidase: A clinical and experimental study. Digestion 1972; 5:326-336

Ikegwuonu FI, Egbunike GN, Emerole GO, Aire TA. The effects of aflatoxin B_1 on some testicular and kidney enzyme activity in rat. Toxicology 1980; 17:9-16

ILAR. Institute of Laboratory Animal Resources, National Research Council, National Academy of Sciences 1980; 64:177-206

Imai S, Morimoto J, Tsubura Y, Hilgers J. Mammary tumor
    virus antigen expression in inbred mouse strains of
    European origin established in Japan. Gann 1980;
    71:419-424

Imamura N, Takahashi T, Lloyd KO, Lewis JL Jr, Old LJ.
    Analysis of human ovarian tumor antigens using heterol-
    ogous antisera: Detection of new antigenic systems. Int
    J Cancer 1978; 21:570-577

Inaba N, Renk T, Wurster K, Rapp W, Bohn H. Ectopic synthe-
    sis of pregnancy specific beta 1-glycoprotein (SP1) and
    placental specific tissue proteins (PP5, PP10, PP11, PP12)
    in nontrophoblastic malignant tumors. Possible markers in
    oncology. Klin Wochenschr 1980; 58:789-791

Ingleton PM, Coulton LA, Preston CJ, Martin TJ. Alkaline
    phosphatase in serum and tumour of rats bearing a hormone-
    responsive transplantable osteogenic sarcoma. Eur J
    Cancer 1979; 15:685-691

Ionescu J, Tapu V, Eskenasy A. Histoenzymology of the lung.
    V. Histoenzymatic analysis of sixty lung tumors. Rev Roum
    MEP 1979; 25:341-348

Irie RF, Irie K, Morton DL. A membrane antigen common to
    human cancer and fetal brain tissues. Cancer Res 1976;
    36:3510-3517

Irving CC. Biochemically detectable tumor markers in urine
    of bladder cancer patients. Cancer Res 1977; 37:2872-2874

Ishikawa S, Kuratomi, Y, Saito T. A case of oat cell carci-
    noma of the lung associated with ectopic production of
    ADH, neurophysin and ACTH. Endocrinol Jpn 1980; 27:257-
    263

Ismail AA, Hamilton JM, Amin AM. Studies of estrogen
    induced renal tumors in male Syrian hamsters. I. Cyto-
    chemical studies of lysosomal enzymes acid phosphatase and
    beta-glucuronidase. Acta Histochem 1978; 61:287-295

Jacobi GH. Laboratory tools in the diagnosis of prostatic
    cancer. Urologe [A] 1979; 18:311-315

Jager G. A simple test for the terminal deoxynucleotidyl
    transferase using the peroxidase-antiperoxidase technique.
    Blut 1981; 42:259-261

Jaken S, Mason M. Differences in the isoelectric focusing
    patterns of gamma-glutamyl transpeptidase from normal and
    cancerous rat mammary tissue. Proc Nat Acad Sci USA 1978;
    75:1750-1753

Jalanko H, Ruoslahti E. Differential expression of α-
    fetoprotein and γ-glutamyltranspeptidase in chemical and
    spontaneous hepatocarcinogenesis. Cancer Res 1979;
    39:3495-3501

Janne J, Poso H, Raina A. Polyamines in rapid growth and
    cancer. Biochim Biophys Acta 1978; 473:241-293

Janossy G, Hoffbrand AV, Greaves MF, Ganishaguru K, Pain C,
    Brandstock KF, Prentice HG, Kay HE, Lister TA. Terminal
    transferase enzyme assay and immunological membrane
    markers in the diagnosis of leukemia: A multiparameter
    analysis of 300 cases. Br J Haematol 1980; 44:221-234

Javadpour N. Serum and cellular biologic tumor markers
    in patients with urologic cancer. Human Pathol 1979; 10:
    557-568

Jensen RK, Sleight SD, Goodman JI, Millis DC, Aust SD,
    Trosko JE. Assessment of the capacity of 3,3',4,4',5,5'-
    hexabromobiphenyl to serve as a promoter of hepatocarcino-
    genesis. Toxicologist 1982; 2:99

Jibiki K, Demura H, Fukunaga T, Yamanaka Y, Hoshino Y.
    Study of serum ferritin in malignant tumors--significance
    as a tumor marker. Horumon to Rinsho 1980; 28:1085-1091

Johnson H, Flye MW, Javadpour N. Serum beta-2-microglobulin
    levels in patients with testicular cancer. Urology 1980;
    16:522-524

Johny KV, Dasgupta MK, Nakashima S, Bossetor JB. Three
    polyethylene glycol dependent methods for the detection
    of circulating immune complexes in pathological sera:
    Comparison with the Raji cell method. J Immunol Methods
    1981; 40:61-71

Jones TC, Hackel DB, Mikagi G. Handbook: Animal Models
    of Human Disease. Washington, DC: Armed Forces Institute
    of Pathology. 1978

Kalengayi MMR, Ronchi G, Desmet VJ. Histochemistry of
    gamma-glutamyl transpeptidase in rat liver during afla-

toxin B$_1$-induced carcinogenesis. J Nat Cancer Inst 1975; 55:579-588

Kallio A, Pösö H, Guha SK, Jänne J. Polyamines and their biosynthetic enzymes in Ehrlich ascites-carcinoma cells. Modification of tumour polyamine pattern by diamines. Biochem J 1977; 166:89-94

Kalwinsky DK, Weatherrel WH, Dahl GV, Bowman WP, Melvin SL, Coleman MS, Bollum FJ. Clinical utility of initial terminal deoxynucleotidyl transferase determinations in childhood acute leukemias. Cancer Res 1981; 41:2877-2881

Kamidono S, Arakawa S, Masuda M, Hamami G, Shimatani N, Itho N, Nakatsuka E, Fujii A, Ohono S, Ishigama J, Yoshimoto Y, Hattori M, Fujita T, Okada S. Significance of measurement of serum levels of tumor markers with germinal cell testicular tumor--value of beta-subunit human chorionic gonadotropin and alpha-fetoprotein. Nippon Hinyokika Gakkai Zasshi 1980; 71:352-362

Kaneko M, Takeuchi T, Tsuchiada Y. Alpha-fetoprotein and other serum proteins synthesized by endodermal sinus tumor transplanted into nude mice. Gann 1980; 71:14-17

Kang YH, West WL. Early response of vaginal epithelium to benzo(a)pyrene in ovariectomized rat: Morphological and cytochemical studies. J Med 1980; 11:169-202

Kanoa K, Honda M, Ishihara S, Ogawa T, Sakata Y, Mastuyuki Y. Clinical application of beta-2-microglobulin measurement in malignant disease. Radioisotopes 1979; 28:459-461

Katopodis N, Hirshaut Y, Geller NL, Stock CC. Lipid-associated sialic acid test for the detection of human cancer. Cancer Res 1982; 42:5270-5275

Katsunuma T, Tsuda M, Kusumi M, Ohkubo T, Mitomi T, Nakasaki H, Tajima T, Yokoyama S, Kamiguchi H, Kobayashi K, Shinoda H. Purification of a serum DNA binding protein (64DP) with a molecular weight of 64,000 and its diagnostic significance in malignant disease. Biochem Biophys Res Commun 1980; 93:552-557

Kawamura N. Staining of bladder tumor cell dehydrogenase. Tokai J Exp Clin Med 1980; 5:421-433

Kelly GJ, Murphy RF, Bridges JM, Elmore DT. An appraisal of phosphatase N as a marker for chronic lymphatic leukemia. Clin Chim Acta 1979; 97:97-99

Kerr DJ, Borek E. The tRNA methyltransferases. Adv Enzymol 1972; 36:1-27

Kersey JH, LeBien TW, Abramson CS, Newman R, Sutherland R, Greaves M. P-24: A human leukemia-associated and lymphohemopoietic progenitor cell surface structure identified with monoclonal antibody. J Exp Med 1981; 153:726-731

Kessel D, Samson MK, Shah P, Allen J, Baker LH. Alterations in plasma sialyltransferase associated with successful chemotherapy of a disseminated tumor. Cancer 1976; 38:2132-2134

Kessel DV, Ratanatharathorn V, Chou TH. Electrofocusing patterns of fucosyltransferases in plasma of patients with neoplastic disease. Cancer Res 1979; 39:3377-3380

Khadapkar SV, Sheth NA, Bhide SV. Independence of sialic acid levels in normal and malignant growth. Cancer Res 1975; 35:1520-1523

Kiesling VI Jr, Watson RA. A closer look at serum prostatic acid phosphatase as a screening test. Urology 1980; 16: 242-244

Kijimoto-Ochiai S, Makita A, Kameya T, Kodama T, Araki E, Yoneyama T. Elevation of glycoprotein galactosyltransferase in human lung cancer related to histological types. Cancer Res 1981; 41:2931-2935

Kim NK, Yasmineh WG, Freier EF, Goldman AI, Theologides A. Value of alkaline phosphatase, 5'-nucleotidase, γ-glutamyltransferase, and glutamate dehydrogenase activity measurements (single and combined) in serum in diagnosis of metastasis to the liver. Clin Chem 1977; 23:2034-2038

Kim YS, Isaacs R. Glycoprotein metabolism in inflammatory and neoplastic diseases of the human colon. Cancer Res 1975; 35:2092-2097

Kirschner MA, Lippman A, Berkowitz R, Mavrer E, Drejka M. Estrogen production as a tumor marker in patients with gonadotropin-producing neoplasms. Cancer Res 1981; 41: 1447-1450

Kitagawa T. Sequential phenotypic changes in hyperplastic areas during hepatocarcinogenesis in the rat. Cancer Res 1976; 36:2534-2539

Kitagawa T, Imai F, Sato K. Re-elevation of gamma-glutamyl transpeptidase activity in periportal hepatocytes of rats with age. Gann 1980a; 71:362-366

Kitagawa T, Pitot HC. The regulation of serine dehydratase and glucose-6-phosphatase in hyperplastic nodules of rat liver during diethylnitrosamine and N-2-fluorenylacetamide feeding. Cancer Res 1975; 35:1075-1084

Kitagawa T, Watanabe R, Sugano H. Induction of gamma-glutamyl transpeptidase activity by dietary phenobarbital in "spontaneous" hepatic tumors of C3H mice. Gann 1980b; 71:536-542

Kitagawa T, Yokochi T, Sugano H. α-Fetoprotein and hepato-carcinogenesis in rats fed 3'-methyl-4-dimethylaminoazo-benzene or N-2-fluorenylacetamide. Int J Cancer 1972; 10:368-381

Klein G. The role of viral transformation and cytogenetic changes in viral oncogenesis. CIBA Found Symp 1979; 66:335-358

Klein G. The role of gene dosage and genetic transpositions in carcinogenesis. Nature 1981; 294:313-318

Klohs WD, Mastrangelo R, Weiser MM. Release of glycosyl-transferase and glycoside activities from normal and transformed cell lines. Cancer Res 1981; 41:2611-2615

Kloppel TM, Morre DJ. Characteristics of transplantable tumors induced in the rat by N-2-fluorenyl-acetamide: Elevations in tissue and serum sialic acid. J Nat Cancer Inst 1980; 64:1401-1411

Kluwe WM. Personal communication. 1981. National Toxicology Program, Research Triangle Park, NC

Knox WE. Enzyme Patterns in Fetal, Adult and Neoplastic Rat Tissues. Basel: S Karger. 1976. p. 231

Koestler TP, Papsidero LD, Nemoto T, Chu TM. Detection of breast tissue-associated antigen by antiserum to Raji cell-bound circulating immune complexes of human breast cancer. Cancer Res 1981; 41:2900-2907

Koett J, Howell J, Wolf PL. Clinical significance of an
ultrafast alkaline phosphatase isoenzyme. J Clin Pathol
1979a; 32:1286-1292

Koett J, Howell J, Wolf PL. The ultrafast alkaline phosphatase isoenzyme is not a bilirubin albumin artifact. Clin
Biochem 1979b; 12:243-245

Köhler G, Milstein C. Continuous cultures of fused cells
secreting antibody of predefined specificity. Nature
1975; 256:495-497

Kojima J, Kanatani M, Nakamura N, Kashiwagi T, Tohjoh F,
Akiyama M. Electrophoretic fractionation of serum gamma-
glutamyl transpeptidase in human hepatic cancer. Clin
Chim Acta 1980a; 106:165-172

Kojima J, Kanatani M, Nakamura N, Kashiwagi T, Tohjoh F,
Akiyama M. Serum and liver glycylproline dipeptidyl
aminopeptidase activity in rats with experimental hepatic
cancer. Clin Chim Acta 1980b; 107:105-110

Kojima J, Kanatani M, Nakamura N, Kashiwagi T, Tohjoh F,
Akiyama M, Tarui Y. Glycylproline dipeptidyl aminopeptidase activities in serum and liver of rats during
3'-methyl DAB administration. Jpn J Gastroenterol 1980c;
77:179-184

Kojima J, Kanatani M, Yamamoto T, Tateishi R, Nakamura N.
Carcinoembryonic proteins in gastric carcinoma metastatic
to the liver. Gastroenterol Jpn 1979; 14:596-603

Kojima S, Hama Y, Kubodera A. Glucose-6-phosphate dehydrogenase and gamma-glutamyltranspeptidase activities in
the liver during chemically induced hepatocarcinogenesis
in rats and mice. Toxicol Appl Pharmacol 1981; 60:26-32

Kollman G, Brennan J. Radioimmunoassay of carcinoembryonic
antigen (CEA) without extraction and dialysis, using solid
phase antibody. J Immunol 1979; 29:387-394

Kondo Y, Sato K, Ueyana Y, Ohsawa N. Serum sialytransferase
and liver datalase activity in cachectic nude mice bearing
a human malignant melanoma. Cancer Res 1981; 41:2912-2926

Korsten CB, Persijn JP, Van der Slik W. The application of
the serum gamma-glutamyl transpeptidase and the 5'-nucleo-
tidase assay in cancer patients: A comparative study.
Z Klin Chem Klin Biochem 1974; 12:116-120

Kouri RE, Billups LH, Rude TH, Whitmire CE, Sass B,
  Henry CJ. Correlation of inducibility of aryl hydrocarbon
  hydroxylase with susceptibility to 3-methylcholanthrene-
  induced lung cancers. Cancer Lett 1980; 9:277-284

Krstulovic AM, Hartwick RA, Brown PR. High performance
  liquid chromatographic determinations of serum UV profiles
  of normal subjects and patients with breast cancer and
  benign fibrocystic changes. Clin Chim Acta 1979; 97:
  159-170

Kuhlmann WD, Krischan R, Kunz W, Guenthner TM, Oesch F.
  Focal elevation of liver microsomal epoxide hydrolase in
  early preneoplastic stages and its behavior in the further
  course of hepatocarcinogenesis. Biochem Biophys Res
  Commun 1981; 98:417-423

Kuhns WJ, Schoentag R. Carcinoma-related alterations of
  glycosyltransferases in human tissues. Cancer Res 1981;
  41:2767-2772

Kuzmits R, Aiginger P, Kuhbok J. Serum fucosyltransferase
  activity in malignant diseases. Acta Med Austriaca Suppl
  1979; 6:349-351

Laishes BA, Ogawa K, Roberts E, Farber E. Gamma-glutamyl
  transpeptidase: A positive marker for cultured rat liver
  cells derived from putative premalignant and malignant
  lesions. J Nat Cancer Inst 1978; 60:1009-1016

Laishes BA, Rolfe PB. Quantitative assessment of liver
  colony formation and hepatocellular carcinoma incidence
  in rats receiving intravenous injections of isogeneic
  liver cells isolated during hepatocarcinogenesis. Cancer
  Res 1980; 40:4133-4143

Lambert PH, Dixon FJ, Zubler RH. A WHO collaborative study
  for the evaluation of eighteen methods of detecting immune
  complexes in serum. J Clin Lab Immunol 1978; 1:1

Lancet Editorial. Immune Complexes in Health and Disease.
  Lancet 1977; i:580-581

Laug WE, Siehel SE, Shaw KN, Landing B, Baptista J,
  Gutenstein M. Initial urinary catecholamine metabolite
  concentrations and prognosis in neuroblastoma. Pediatrics
  1978; 62:77-83

Laurent G, Doriaux M, Hildebrand J. Isolation of plasma membranes from murine ependymoblastoma and subcellular distribution of amphotericin B in this tumor. Biochim Biophys Acta 1977; 466:123-135

Leboy PS, Glick JM. tRNA methyltransferases from rat liver. Differences in response of partially purified enzymes to polyamines and inorganic salts. Biochim Biophys Acta 1976; 435:30-38

Leder P, Konkel D, Leder A, Nishioka Y. Globin genes: A paradigm of gene structure, function and evolution. Nat Cancer Inst Monogr 1982; 60:49-54

Lee C, Murphy GP, Chu TM. Purification and characterization of acid phosphatase from Dunning R3327h prostatic adeno-carcinoma. Cancer Res 1980c; 40:1245-1248

Lee IP, Suzuki K, Lee SD, Dixon RL. Aryl hydrocarbon hydroxylase induction in rat lung, liver, and male repro-ductive organs following inhalation exposure to diesel emission. Toxicol Appl Pharmacol 1980b; 52:181-184

Lee JN, Salem HT, Al-Ani AT, Chard T, Huang SC, Duyang PC, Wei PY, Seppala M. Circulating concentrations of specific placental proteins (human chorionic gonadotropin, preg-nancy-specific beta-1 glycoprotein, and placental protein 5) in untreated gestational trophoblastic tumors. Am J Obstet Gynecol 1981; 139:702-704

Lee YT, Tokes ZA, Csipke CP. Plasma sialyltransferase in patients with breast cancer. J Surg Oncol 1980a; 14:159-165

Leffert HL, Moran T, Boorstein R, Koch KS. PPO carcinogen activation and hormonal control of cell proliferation in differentiated primary adult rat liver cell cultures. Nature (London) 1977; 267:58-61

Lei-Injo LE, Tsou KC, Lo KW, Lopez CG, Balasegaram M, Ganesan S. 5'-Nucleotide phosphodiesterase isozyme-V in health, in cancer, and in viral hepatitis. Cancer 1980; 45:795-798

Lerman MI, Abaskumova OY, Kucenco NG, Gorbacheva LB, Kukushkina GV, Serebryanyi AM. Different degradation rates of alkylated RNA protein and lipids in normal and tumor cells. Cancer Res 1974; 34:1536-1541

Lerner MP, Anglin JH, Norquist RE. Cell-surface antigens
from human breast tumor cells. J Nat Cancer Inst 1978;
60:39-44

Leung JP, Bordin GM, Nakamura RM, DeHeer DH, Edgington TS.
Frequency of association of mammary tumor glycoprotein
antigen and other markers with human breast tumors.
Cancer Res 1979; 39:2057-2061

Leung JP, Edgington TS. Subcellular localization of the
sedimentable form of mammary tumor glycoprotein to the
tumor cell plasmalemma. Cancer Res 1980; 40:316-321

Leveson SH, Howell JH, Holyoke ED, Goldrosen MH. Leukocyte
adherence inhibition: An automated microassay demonstrating specific antigen recognition and blocking activity in
two murine tumor systems. J Immunol Methods 1977; 17:
153-162

Levine AM, Rosenberg SA. Alkaline phosphatase levels in
osteosarcoma tissue are related to prognosis. Cancer
1979; 44:2291-2293

Levine L, Waalkes TP, Stolbach L. Serum levels of N^2, N^2-
dimethylguanosine and pseudouridine as determined by
radioimmunoassay for patients with malignancy. J Nat
Cancer Inst 1975; 54:341-343

Levinson AD, Oppermann H, Levintow L, Varmus HE, Bishop JM.
Evidence that the transforming gene of ovarian sarcoma
virus encodes a protein kinase associated with a phospho-
protein. Cell 1978; 15:561-72

Lewkonia RM, Kerr EJ, Irvine WJ. Clinical evaluation of the
macrophage electrophoretic mobility test for cancer. Br J
Cancer 1974; 30:532-537

Lin CW, Inglis NR, Rule AH, Turksoy RN, Chapman CM,
Kirley SD, Stolbach II. Histaminase and other tumor
markers in malignant effusion fluids. Cancer Res 1979;
39:4894-4899

Linder MC, Bryant RR, Lim S, Scott LE, Moor JE. Ceruloplasmin elevation and synthesis in rats with transplantable
tumors. Enzyme 1979; 24:85-95

Linder MC, Munro HN. Metabolic and chemical features of
ferritins, a series of iron-inducible tissue proteins.
Am J Pathol 1973; 72:263-282

Lipkin M. Phase I and Phase II proliferative lesions of colonic epithelial cells in diseases leading to colonic cancer. Cancer 1974; 34:878-888

Lipsky MM, Hinton DE, Klaunig JE, Goldblatt PJ, Trump BF. Biology of hepatocellular neoplasia in the mouse. II. Sequential enzyme histochemical analysis of BALB/c mouse liver during safrole-induced carcinogenesis. J Nat Cancer Inst 1981; 67:377-392

Lisiewicz J, Gierek T, Pilch J. Deficiency of beta-glucuronidase in neutrophiles from patients with precancerous states of the larynx. Folia Haematol 1978; 105:194-199

Lisiewicz J, Gierek T, Pilch J, Piastucka B. The enzymatic equipment of neutrophils in patients with precancerous states of the larynx. Med Interne 1978; 16:33-36

Litt M. Heterogeneity of turnover rates of 4S RNAs in Friend virus infected mouse leukemia cells. Biochem Biophys Res Commun 1975; 66:658-664

Liu CK, Schmied R, Waxman S. The specific release of sialyltransferase activity by human hepatoma cell lines. Clin Chim Acta 1979; 98:225-233

Lloyd KO. Human ovarian tumor antigens. In: Serologic Analysis of Human Cancer Antigens. New York: Academic Press. 1980. pp. 515-526

Lloyd KO, Ng J, Dippold WG. Analysis of the biosynthesis of HLA-DR glycoproteins in human malignant melanoma cell lines. J Immunol 1981; 126:2408-2413

Loewenstein PM, Lange GW, Gerard GF. Distribution of DNA polymerase Cm in normal and malignant human tissues. Cancer Res 1980; 40:4398-4402

Logan J, Cairns J. The secrets of cancer. Nature 1982; 300:104-105

LoGerfo P, Krupey J, Hansen HJ. Demonstration of an antigen common to several varieties of neoplasia. New Engl J Med 1971; 285:138-141

Lokich JJ. Tumor markers: Hormones, antigens, and enzymes in malignant disease. Oncology 1978; 35:54-57

Lombardi B, Shinozuka H.   Enhancement of 2-acetylamino-
fluorene liver carcinogenesis in rats fed a choline-devoid
diet.   Int J Cancer 1979; 23:565-570

Long JC, McCaffrey RP, Aisenberg AC.   Terminal deoxynucleotidyl transferase positive lymphoblastic lymphoma.   A
study of 15 cases.   Cancer 1979; 44:2127-2139

Lorenz J, Schassmann H, Ohnhaus E, Oesch F.   Activities of
polycyclic hydrocarbon activating and inactivating enzymes
in human lungs of smokers, non-smokers, lung-cancer and
non-cancer patients.   Arch Toxicol 1979; 41:483-489

Lukes RJ, Collins RD.   New approaches to the classification
of the lymphomata.   Br J Cancer 1975; 31:1-28

Lynch HT, Thomas RH, Terasaki PI, Ting A, Guirgis HA, Kaplan
AR, Magee H, Lynch J, Kraft C, Chaperon E.   HL-A in cancer
family "N."   Cancer 1975; 36:1315

Mabuchi M.   Sequential hepatic changes during sterigmato-
cystin-induced carcinogenesis in the rat.   Jpn J Exp Med
1979; 49:365-372

Malkin A, Kellen JA, Lickrish GM, Bush RS.   Carcinoembryonic
antigen (CEA) and other tumor markers in ovarian and cervical cancer.   Cancer 1978; 42:1452-1456

Maluish AE.   Experiences with leukocyte adherence inhibition
in human cancer.   Cancer Res 1979; 39:644-648

Mandel LR, Srinivasan PR, Borek E.   Origin of urinary methylated purines.   Nature 1966; 209:586-588

Maor D, Mardiney MR Jr.   Alteration of human serum ribonuclease activity in malignancy.   CRC Crit Rev Clin Lab
Sci 1978; 10:89-111

Marcus DM, Zinberg N.   Measurement of serum ferritin by
radioimmunoassay: Results in normal individuals and
patients with breast cancer.   J Nat Cancer Inst 1975;
55:791-795

Marks PA.   Genetically determined susceptibility to cancer.
Blood 1981; 58:415-419

Marshall MJ, Neal FE, Goldberg DM.   Isoenzymes of hexokinase, 6-phosphogluconate dehydrogenase, phosphoglucomutase

and lactate dehydrogenase in uterine cancer. Br J Cancer 1979; 40:380-390

Marton LJ. CSF polyamines: Potential as brain tumor markers. Arch Neurol 1981; 38:73-74

Marton LJ, Edwards MS, Levin VA, Lubich WP, Wilson CB. CSF polyamines: A new and important means of monitoring patients with medulloblastoma. Cancer 1981; 47:757-760

Matsui I, Otani S, Morisawa S. Effect of urethane on polyamine and DNA synthesis in the regenerating rat liver. Chem Biol Interact 1980; 30:35-43

Matsukura N, Kinebuchi M, Kawachi T, Sato S, Sugimura T. Quantitative measurement of intestinal marker enzymes in intestinal metaplasia from human stomach with cancer. Gann 1979; 70:509-513

Matsushima M, Bryan GT. Early induction of mouse urinary bladder ornithine decarboxylase activity of rodent vesical carcinogens. Cancer Res 1980; 1897-1901

Mattenheimer H. Enzymes in renal diseases. Ann Clin Lab Sci 1977; 7:422-432

Max EE, Battey J, Ney R, Kirsch IR, Leder P. Duplication and deletion in the human immunoglobulin epsilon genes. Cell 1982; 29:691-699

Maxim PE, Veltri RW, Sprinkle PM. Soluble tumor-associated markers in lung cancer extracts. Oncology 1981; 38: 147-153

McCaffrey R, Lillquist A, Sallan S, Cohen E, Osband M. Clinical utility of leukemia cell terminal transferase measurements. Cancer Res 1981; 41:4814-4820

McCartney WR, Hoffer PB. The value of carcinoembryonic antigen (CEA) as an adjunct to the radiological colon examination in the diagnosis of malignancy. Radiology 1974; 110:325-328

McCoy JL, Dean JH, Cannon GB, Jerome LJ, Alford TC, Parks WP, Gilden RV, Oroszlan ST, Herberman RB. Leukocyte migration inhibition and lymphocyte blastogenesis responses in breast carcinoma patients to mouse mammary tumor virus and to virion gp52 antigen and Rauscher murine

leukemia virus-Kirsten sarcoma virus gp69/71 antigen.
J Nat Cancer Inst 1978; 60:1259-1267

McCoy JL, Jerome LF, Anderson C, Cannon GB, Alford TC,
    Connor RJ, Oldham RK, Herberman RB. Leukocyte migration
    inhibition by soluble extracts of MDF-7 tissue culture
    cell line derived from breast carcinoma. J Nat Cancer
    Inst 1976; 57:1045-1049

McGee JO, Woods JC, Ashall F, Bramwell ME, Harris H. A
    new marker for human cancer cells. 2. Immunohistochemical
    detection of the Ca antigen in human tissues with the Ca1
    antibody. Lancet 1982; 8288:7-10

McIntire KR, Greenberg LP. Carcinoembryonic antigen:
    Its role as a marker in the management of cancer (National
    Institutes of Health Concensus Development Conference
    Statement). Cancer Res 1981; 41:2017-2018

Meierhenry EF, Ruebner BH, Gershwin ME, Hsieh LS, French
    SW. Mallory body formation in hepatic nodules of mice
    ingesting dieldrin. Lab Invest 1981; 44:392-396

Meister A. Glutathione and the γ-glutamyl cycle. In:
    Glutathione: Metabolism and Function. Aris IM,
    Jakoby WB. eds. New York: Raven Press. 1976.
    pp. 35-43

Melnick JL, Adam E, Lewis R, Kaufman RH. Cervical cancer
    cell lines containing herpes virus markers. Intervirology
    1979; 12:111-114

Michael SC, Taguchi O, Nishizuka Y. Changes in hypophyseal
    hormones associated with accelerated aging and tumorigene-
    sis of the ovaries in neonatally thymectomized mice.
    Endocrinology 1981; 108:2375-2380

Micheau C, Bernard A, Pujade E, Belpomme D, Carlu C,
    Clausse B. Non-Hodgkin's malignant lymphoma: Reliability
    of "typing" using cyto-enzymatic markers. Comparison with
    immunological markers. Nouv Presse Med 1980; 9:167-170

Michelson JB, Felberg NT, Shields JA. Evaluation of meta-
    static cancer to the eye. Carcinoembryonic antigen and
    gamma glutamyl transpeptidase. Arch Ophthalmol 1977;
    95:692-694

Miki K, Oda T, Miyazaki J, Iino S, Niwa H, Oka H, Suzuki S.
    Alkaline phosphatase isoenzymes in intestinal metaplasia

and carcinoma of rat stomach induced by N-methyl-N'-nitro-N-nitrosoguanidine. Oncodev Biol Med 1980; 1:313-323

Milano G, Aussel C, Stora C, Lafaurie M, Stoula G, Lalanne C. Intrahepatic polyamine levels during rat liver carcinogenesis induced by N-2-fluorenylacetamide. Carcinogenesis 1981; 2:109-114

Milhaud G, Calmettes C, Jullienne A, Ribeiro F, Moukhtar MS. Calcitonin (in cancer). Int Congr Ser-Excerpta Med 1977; 403:430-436

Mitsuyama T. Experimental and clinical studies on ribose-phosphate isomerase. Hokkaido Igaku Zassshi 1979; 54: 387-400

Mizejewski GJ, Allen RP. Immuno therapeutic suppression in transplantable solid tumors. Nature (London) 1974; 250: 50-52

Mod A, Carpentier N, Füst G, Lambert PH, Miescher P, Hollan SR. Serial measurement of circulating immune complexes in the sera of patients with leukemia. J Clin Lab Immunol 1980; 4:15-20

Modak MJ, Mortelsmann R, Kozimer B, Pahwa R, Moore MA, Clarkson BD, Good RA. A micromethod for determination of terminal deoxynucleotidyl transferase (TdT) in the diagnostic evaluation of acute leukemias. J Cancer Res Clin Oncol 1980; 98:91-104

Montesano R, Bannikov G, Drevon C, Kuroki T, Saint Vincent L, Tomatis L. Neoplastic transformation of rat liver epithelial cells in cultures. Ann NY Acad Sci 1980; 349:323-331

Moore MR, Drinkwater NR, Miller EC, Miller JA, Pitot HC. Quantitative analysis of the time-dependent development of glucose-6-phosphatase-deficient foci in the livers of mice treated neonatally with diethylnitrosamine. Cancer Res 1981; 41:1585-1593

Moossa AR, Levin B. The diagnosis of "early" pancreatic cancer: The University of Chicago experience. Cancer 1981; 47:1688-1697

Moretta L. In: Immunology 80. Fougereau M, Dausset J. eds. New York: Academic Press. 1980. p. 223

Morgan RW, Ward JM, Hartman PE. Detection of mutagens-carcinogens: Carcinogen-induced lesions pinpointed by alkaline phosphatase activity in fixed gastric specimens from rats. J Nat Cancer Inst 1981; 66:941-945

Moser K, Dorner F, Francesconi M, Ganzinger U, Graninger W, Lenzhofer R, Pesendorfer FX, Pohl A, Rainer H. Developments in the serological diagnosis of malignant diseases. Wien Klin Wochenschr 1980; 92:789-796

Motomiya Y, Yamada K, Matsushima S, Ijyuin M, Iriya K. Studies on urinary isozymes of lactic dehydrogenase and beta-glucuronidase in patients with bladder tumors. Urol Res 1975; 3:41-48

Mrochek JE, Dinsmore SR, Tormey DC, Waalkes TP. Protein-bound carbohydrates in breast cancer. Liquid-chromatographic analysis for mannose, galactose, fucose and sialic acid in serum. Clin Chem 1976; 22:1516-1521

Mrochek JE, Dinsmore SR, Waalkes TP. Analytical techniques in the separation and identification of specific purine and pyrimidine degradation products of tRNA: Application to urine samples from cancer patients. J Nat Cancer Inst 1974; 53:1553-1563

Mrochek JE, Dinsmore SR, Waalkes TP. Liquid chromatographic analysis for neutral carbohydrates in serum glycoproteins. Clin Chem 1975; 21:1314

Mullen JL, Pollock TW, Tsou KC, Lo KW, Rosato EF. Detection of hepatic metastases with serum 5'-nucleotide phosphodiesterase. Surg Form 1976; 27:107-108

Müller R, Rajewsky MF. Immunological quantification by high-affinity antibodies of O^6-ethyldeoxyguanosine in DNA exposed to N-ethyl-N-nitrosourea. Cancer Res 1980; 40: 887-896

Murphy GR. ed. Models for prostate cancer. In: Proceedings, Progress in Clinical and Biological Research Series. New York: Alan R. Liss, Inc. 1980

Murphy SB. Childhood non-Hodgkin's lymphoma. New Engl J Med 1978; 299:1446-1448

Nagarajan B, Sukumar S. Changes in polyamine content during hepatocarcinogenesis. Indian J Cancer 1979; 15:55-59

NAS. National Academy of Sciences. Committee for the Revision of NAS Publication 1138. Principles and procedures for evaluating the toxicity of household substances. Washington DC: National Academy of Sciences. 1977

Nathanson L, Fishman WH. New observations on the Regan isoenzyme of alkaline phosphatase in cancer patients. Cancer 1971; 27:1388-1397

National Center for Health Statistics. Monthly vital statistics report, Vol. 30, No. 11. February 10, 1982. pp. 8-9

National Institutes of Health. Surveillance, epidemiology, and end results: Incidence and mortality data, 1973-77. National Cancer Institute Monograph 57, NIH Publ. No. 81-2330. Bethesda MD: U.S. Department of Health and Human Services. 1981

Nemoto T, Constantine R, Chu TM. Human tissue polypeptide antigen in breast cancer. J Nat Cancer Inst 1979; 63: 1347-1350

Nery R, Neville AM. Cancer indicating substances in urine. Science Foundation Urology Conference Proceedings. London: Heineman Medical Books. 1976. pp. 215-221

Neumann H, Klein E, Hauck-Granoth R, Yachnin S, Ben-Bassat H. Comparative study of alkaline phosphatase activity in lymphocytes, mitogen-induced blasts, lymphoblastoid cell lines, acute myeloid leukemia, and chronic lymphatic leukemia cells. Proc Nat Acad Sci USA 1976; 73:1432-1436

Neuwald PD, Anderson C, Salivar WO, Aldenderfer PH, Dermody WC, Weintraub BD, Rosen SW, Nelson-Rees WA, Ruddon RW. Expression of oncodevelopmental gene products by human tumor cells in culture. J Nat Cancer Inst 1980; 64:447-459

Neuwald PD, Brooks M. Altered form of placental alkaline phosphatase produced by JAR choriocarcinoma cells in culture. Cancer Res 1981; 41:1682-1689

Neville AM, Coombes RC, Hillyard CJ, MacIntyre I. Calcitonin as a tumor marker. In: Cancer Related Antigens: Symposium. Franchimont P. ed. Amsterdam: North-Holland. 1976. pp. 151-162

Nicolson GL. Lectin interactions with normal and tumor cells and affinity purification of cell glycoproteins. In: Cancer Markers: Diagnostic and Developmental Significance. Sell S. ed. Clifton NJ: Humana Press. 1980. pp. 403-443.

Nievel JG, Anderson J, Bray P. Biochemical changes in liver and blood underlying parenchymal damage of rat liver induced by a dose-dependent effect of drugs before and after development of liver enlargement and nodular hyperplasia. Biochem Soc Trans 1976; 4:932-933

Niinobe M, Tamura Y, Arima T, Fujii S. Immunological properties of and neuraminidase action on aminopeptidases and arylamidases in human normal and cancer tissues. Cancer Res 1979; 39:4212-4217

Nishida K, Kondo M, Jessen K, Classen M. Diagnosis of pancreatic cancer by pancreatic oncofetal antigen (POA) in pure pancreatic juice. Hepato-Gastroenterol 1981; 28:102-105

Nishimura S, Kuchino Y. Transfer RNA and cancer. Gann Monogr Cancer Res 1979; 24:245-262

Nishioka K, Ezaki K, Hart JS. A preliminary study of polyamines in the bone-marrow plasma of adult patients with leukemia. Clin Chim Acta 1980; 107:59-66

Nomura Y. Biological evidence for possibility of the intracellular mechanism scavenging deformed tRNA molecules. FEBS Lett 1974; 45:223-227

Nordquist RE, Anglin JH, Lerner MP. Antigen shedding by human breast-cancer cells in vitro and in vivo. Br J Cancer 1978; 37:776-779

Norpoth K, Gottschalk D, Gottschalk I, Witting U, Thomas H, Eichner D, Schmidt EH. Influence of vinyl chloride monomer (VCM) and As 203 on rat liver cell proliferation after partial hepatectomy. J Cancer Res Clin Oncol 1980; 97:41-50

Novikoff AB, Novikoff PM, Stockert RJ, Becker FF, Yam A, Poruchynsky MS, Levin W, Thomas PE. Immunocytochemical localization of epoxide hydrase in hyperplastic nodules induced in rat liver by 2-acetylaminofluorene. Proc Nat Acad Sci USA 1979; 76:5207-5211

Novogrodsky A, Tate SS, Meister A. Gamma-glutamyl transpeptidase, a lymphoid cell-surface marker: Relationship to
blastogenesis, differentiation, and neoplasia. Proc Nat
Acad Sci USA 1976; 73:2414-2418

NTP. National Toxicology Program. Fiscal year 1982, annual
plan. Washington DC: Department of Health and Human
Services, U.S. Public Health Service. March 1982

Nydeggar UE, Lambert PH, Gerber H, Miescher PA. Circulating
immune complexes in the serum in systemic lupus erythematosus and in cancers of the hepatitis B antigens. Quantitation by binding to radiolabeled Clq. J Clin Invest
1974; 54:279-309

O'Brien MJ, Kirkham SE, Burke B, Ormerod M, Saravis CA,
Gottleib LS, Neville AM, Zamcheck N. CEA, ZGM and EMA
localization in cells of pleural and peritoneal effusion:
A preliminary study. Invest Cell Pathol 1980; 3:251-258

Odani S, Sakamoto S, Yachi A. Studies on serum protein
changes during 3'-methyl-4-dimethylaminoazobenzene hepatocarcinogenesis in rats. I. Comparative studies on serum
proteins, especially seromucoid and haptoglobin in alpha-
fetoprotein. Sapporo Med J 1980; 49:187-203

Odell W, Wolfsen A, Yoshimoto Y, Weitzman R, Fisher D,
Hirose F. Ectopic peptide synthesis: A universal concomitant of neoplasia. Trans Assoc Am Physicians 1977;
90:204-227

Ogawa K, Onoe T, Takeuchi M. Spontaneous occurrence of γ-
glutamyl transpeptidase-positive hepatocytic foci in 105-
week-old Wistar and 72-week-old Fischer 344 male rats.
J Nat Cancer Inst 1981; 67:407-412

Ogawa K, Solt DB, Farber E. Phenotypic diversity as an
early property of putative preneoplastic hepatocyte populations in liver carcinogenesis. Cancer Res 1980; 40:725-
733

Ohde G, Schuppler J, Schulte-Hermann R, Keiger H. Proliferation of rat liver cells in preneoplastic nodules after
stimulation of liver growth by xenobiotic inducers. Arch
Toxicol 1979; 41:451-455

Ohmori T, Rice JM, Williams GM. Histochemical characteristics of spontaneous and chemically induced hepatocellular
neoplasms in mice and the development of neoplasms with

gamma-glutamyltranspeptidase activity during phenobarbital exposure. Histochem J 1981; 13:85-99

Ohno T, Mesa-Tejada R, Keydar I, Ramanarayanan M, Bausch J, Spiegelman S. Human breast carcinoma antigen is immunologically related to the polypeptide of the group-specific glycoprotein of mouse mammary tumor virus. Proc Nat Acad Sci 1979; 76:2460-2464

Oh-Uti K, Inoue S, Minato S. Purification of an anemia-inducing factor from human placenta and its application to diagnosis of malignant neoplasms. Cancer Res 1980; 40:1686-1690

Okamura S, Crane F, Jamal N. Single-cell immunofluorescence assay for terminal transferase: Human leukemic and non-leukemic cells. Br J Cancer 1980; 41:159-167

Okita K, Farber E. An antigen common to preneoplastic hepatocyte populations and to liver cancer induced by N-2-fluorenyl-acetamide, ethionine or other hepatocarcinogens. Gann 1975; 17:283-299

Olson JW, Russell DH. Prolonged ornithine decarboxylase induction in regenerating carcinogen-treated liver. Cancer Res 1980; 40:4373-4380

Oncology Overview--Selected Abstracts on Pancreatic Carcinogenesis, USDHEW. 1980

Onoe T, Empo K, Kaneko A. Significance of α-fetoprotein appearance in the early stage of azo-dye carcinogenesis. Gann 1973; 14:233-243

Oon CJ, Yo Sui Lan. Presence of a hepatoma-liver antigen in the sera of patients with primary hepatocellular carcinoma. Singapore Med J 1979; 20:317-322

Order SE, Klein JL. The utilization of antigens in ovarian cancer. In: Serologic Analysis of Human Cancer Antigens. Rosenberg SA. ed. New York: Academic Press. 1980. pp. 527-537

Order SE, Rosenshein NB, Klein JL, Lichter AS, Ettinger DS, Dillon MB, Leibel SA. New methods applied to the analysis and treatment of ovarian cancer. Int J Radiat Oncol Biol Phys 1979; 5:861-873

Orlando M, Ceccarini M, Hassan HJ, Longo M, Annino L. Electrophoretic pattern of non-specific esterases in normal subjects and cases of chronic granulocytic leukemia. IRCS Med Sci 1980; 8:362

Oshiumi Y, Yagi H, Nishitani H, Yamawaki H, Nakayana C, Kamoi I, Matsuura K, Momose S. Clinical significance of urinary CEA measurements as a screening test of bladder cancer. Radioisotopes 1979; 28:367-370

Oyanagui Y, Sato N, Hagihara B. Spectrophotometric analysis of cytochromes in rat liver during carcinogenesis. Cancer Res 1974; 34:458-462

Panfili PR. Mouse lymphocyte differentiation markers. In: Cancer Markers: Diagnostic and Developmental Significance. Sell S. ed. Clifton NJ: Humana Press. 1980. pp. 37-55

Pangalis GA, Bentler E. Terminal transferase in leukemia of adults. Acta Haematol 1979; 62:199-205

Paone JF, Waalkes TP, Baker RR, Shaper JH. Serum UDP-galactosyltransferase as a potential biomarker for breast carcinoma. J Surg Oncol 1980; 15:59-66

Papsidero LD, Nemoto T, Snyderman MC, Chu TM. Immune complexes in breast cancer patients as detected by C1q binding. Cancer 1979; 44:1636-1640

Pearson G, Freeman G. Evidence suggesting a relationship between polyoma virus-induced transplantation antigen and normal embryonic antigen. Cancer Res 1968; 28:1665-1673

Pepersack L, Lee JC, McEwan R, Ihle JH. Phenotypic heterogenicity of Maloney leukemia virus induced T cell lymphomas. J Immunol 1980; 124:279-285

Peraino C, Fry RJ, Staffeldt E. Reduction and enhancement by phenobarbital of hepatocarcinogenesis induced in the rat by 2-acetylaminofluorene. Cancer Res 1971; 31:1056-1112

Peraino C, Fry RJ, Staffeldt E. Effects of varying the onset and duration of exposure to phenobarbital on its enhancement of 2-acetylaminofluorene-induced hepatic tumorigenesis. Cancer Res 1977; 37:3623-3627

Peraino C, Fry RJ, Staffeldt E, Christopher JP. Comparative enhancing effects of phenobarbital, amobarbital, diphenyl-hydantoin, and dichlorodiphenyl-trichloroethane on 2-acetylaminofluorene-induced hepatic tumorigenesis in the rat. Cancer Res 1975; 35:2884-2890

Peraino C, Staffeldt EF, Ludeman VA. Early appearance of histochemically altered hepatocyte foci and liver tumors in female rats treated with carcinogens one day after birth. Carcinogenesis 1981; 2:463-465

Pereira MA. Rat liver foci bioassay. J Am Coll Toxicol 1982; 1:101-117

Pich A, Bussolati G, Carbonara A. Immunocytochemical detection of casein and casein-like proteins in human tissues. J Histochem Cytochem 1976; 24:940-947

Pichler WJ, Broder S. Fc-IgM and Fc-IgG receptors on human circulating B lymphocytes. J Immunol 1978; 121:887-890

Pietras RJ, Szego CM, Mangan CE, Seeler BJ, Burtnett MM, Orevi M. Elevated serum cathepsin B1 and vaginal pathology after prenatal DES exposure. Obstet Gynecol 1978; 52:321-327

Pitot HC. The natural history of neoplasia. Am J Pathol 1977; 89:402-412

Pitot HC, Barsness L, Goldsworthy T, Kitagawa T. Biochemical characterization of stages of hepatocarcinogenesis after a single dose of diethylnitrosamine. Nature 1978; 271:456-458

Pitot HC, Goldsworthy T, Campbell HA, Poland A. Quantitative evaluation of the promotion by 2,3,7,8-tetrachlorodibenzo-p-dioxin of hepatocarcinogenesis from diethylnitrosamine. Cancer Res 1980; 40:3616-3620

Pitot HC, Sirica AE. The stages of initiation and promotion in hepatocarcinogenesis. Biochim Biophys Acta 1980; 605:191-215

Platt DS, Cockrill BL. Biochemical changes in rat liver in response to treatment with drugs and other agents. III. Effects of centrally acting drugs. Biochem Pharmacol 1969; 18:459-473

Podolsky DK, Isselbacher KJ. Cancer-associated galactosyltransferase acceptor: Inhibition of transformed cell and
  tumor growth. Cancer Suppl 1980; 45:1212-1217

Podolsky DK, McPhee MS, Alpert E, Warshaw AL,
  Isselbacher KJ. Galactosyltransferase isoenzyme II in
  the detection of pancreatic cancer: Comparison with
  radiologic, endoscopic and serologic tests. New Engl J
  Med 1981; 304:1313-1318

Podolsky DK, Weiser MM. Galactosyltransferase activities
  in human sera: Detection of a cancer associated isoenzyme. Biochem Biophys Res Commun 1975; 65:545-551

Podolsky DK, Weiser MM. Purification of galactosyltransferase isoenzymes I and II. Comparison of cancer associated
  and normal galactosyltransferase activities. J Biol Chem
  1979; 254:3983-3990

Podolsky DK, Weiser MM, Isselbacher KJ, Cohen AM. A cancer-
  associated galactosyltransferase isoenzyme. New Engl J
  Med 1978; 299:703-705

Podolsky DK, Weiser MM, Westwood JC, Gammon M. Cancer-
  associated serum galactosyltransferase demonstration in
  an animal model system. J Biol Chem 1977; 252:1807-1813

Pohl A, Moser K. A galactosyltransferase isoenzyme as a
  tumor specific diagnostic aid. Verh Dtsch Ges Inn Med
  1978; pp. 594-597

Poirier MC. Antibodies to carcinogen-DNA adducts. J Nat
  Cancer Inst 1981; 67:515-519

Pollard M, Luckert PH, Schmidt MA. Production of prostatic
  adenocarcinoma in Lobund Wistar rats by testosterone. The
  Prostate 1983 (in press)

Pollock TW, Mullen JL, Tsou KC, Lo W, Rosato EF. Serum 5'-
  nucleotide phosphodiesterase as a predictor of hepatic
  metastases in gastrointestinal cancer. Am J Surg 1979;
  137:22-25

Pompecki R, Winkler R. Clinical significance of routine
  serum CEA determination in postoperative control in
  colorectal cancer. Med Welt 1980; 31:1780-1783

Poole AR, Tiltman KJ, Recklies AD, Stoker TA. Differences in secretion of the proteinase cathepsin B at the edges of human breast carcinomas and fibroadenomas. Nature 1978; 273:545-547

Poppema S, Elema JD, Halie MR. Alkaline phosphatase positive lymphomas: A morphologic, immunologic, and enzymehistochemical study. Cancer 1981; 47:1303-1312

Posey LE, Rainey J, Vial R, Ryan D, Bickers JH, Morgan LR, Samuels MS, Hull EW. A noninvasive technique for monitoring response to chemotherapy in human acute leukemia. Cancer 1979; 44:873-880

Posner JB. Cerebrospinal fluid biochemical markers of central nervous system metastasis. Ann Neurol 1980; 8:597-604

Potter TP Jr, Lasater HA, Jordan TA, Jordan JD, Johnston RK, Oishi N. Tennessee antigen--clinical application. Cancer Detect Prev 1980; 3

Pradhan SL, Dixit CV, Shah AK. The diagnostic significance of serum fucose in various malignant diseases. Indian J Pathol Microbiol 1979; 22:21-26

Preud'Homme JL, Seligmann M. In: Progress in Clinical Immunology. Schwartz RS. ed. New York: Grune and Stratton. 1974. p. 121

Procházka J, Deyl Z, Havránek T, Grafouá E, Janatková I, Stulíková V, Sobeslavský C. Discrimination analysis as a tool for classifying the value of biochemical and immunological tests in lung cancer. Oncology 1981; 38:230-235

Pugh TD, Goldfarb S. Quantitative histochemical and auto-radiographic studies of hepatocarcinogenesis in rats fed 2-acetylaminofluorene followed by phenobarbital. Cancer Res 1978; 38:4450-4457

Pulay TA, Csömör A. Tumor differentiation and immunocom-petence in cervical cancer patients. Neoplasma 1979; 26: 617-621

Pullicino P, Thompson EJ, Moseley IF, Zilkha E, Shortman RC. Cystic intracranial tumours. Cyst fluid, biochemical changes and computerised tomographic findings. J Neurol Sci 1979; 44:77-85

Rady P, Arany I, Bojan F, Kertai P. Activities of four
glycolytic enzymes (HK, PFK, PK_1 and LDH) and isozymic
pattern of LDH in mouse lung tumor induced by urethan.
J Cancer Res Clin Oncol 1979; 95:287-289

Rady P, Arany I, Bojan F, Kertai P. Effect of carcinogenic
and noncarcinogenic chemicals on the activities of four
glycolytic enzymes in mouse lung. Chem Biol Interact
1980; 31:209-213

Randerath E, Copalakrishnan AS, Gupta RC, Agrwal HP,
Randerath K. Lack of a specific ribose methylation at
guanosine 17 in Morris hepatoma 5123D $tRNA_{IBA}^{Ser1}$. Cancer
Res 1981; 41:2863-2867

Rao MS, Lalwani ND, Scarpelli DG, Reddy JK. The absence
of γ-glutamyl transpeptidase activity in putative preneoplastic lesions and in hepatocellular carcinomas induced
in rats by the hypolipidemic peroxisome proliferator Wy-
14,643. Carcinogenesis 1982; 3:1231-1233.

Rao KN, Takahashi S, Shinozuka H. Acinar cell carcinoma of
the rat pancreas grown in cell culture and in nude mice.
Cancer Res 1980; 40:592-597

Rasmussen RE, Boyd CH, Dansie DR, Kouri RE, Henry CJ. DNA
replication and unscheduled DNA synthesis in lungs of mice
exposed to cigarette smoke. Cancer Res 1981; 41:2583-2588

Rattanapanone V, Tashiro S, Tikuda H, Rattanapanone N,
Ito Y. Cellular retinoic acid binding protein in virus-
induced Shope papillomas of rabbit skin. Cancer Res 1981;
41:1483-1487

Reaman GH, Blatt J, Poplack DG, Bagley CM. Independence of
purine pathway enzyme abnormalities in acute lymphoblastic
leukemia (ALL). Proc Am Assoc Cancer Res 1981; 22:320

Reddi KK, Holland JF. Elevated serum ribonuclease in
patients with pancreatic cancer. Proc Nat Acad Sci USA
1976; 73:2308-2310

Reddy EP, Reynolds RK, Santos E, Barbacid M. A point mutation is responsible for the acquisition of transforming
properties by the T24 human bladder carcinoma oncogene.
Nature 1982; 300:149-152

Rees LH. The biosynthesis of hormones by non-endocrine
tumors--a review. J Endocrinol 1975; 67:143-175

Reinherz EL, Nadler LM, Rosenthal DS, Moloney WC, Schlossman SF. T-cell-subset characterization of human T-CLL. Blood 1979; 53:1066-1075

Reintoft I, Hagerstrand I. Demonstration of α_1-antitrypsin in hepatomas. Arch Pathol Lab Med 1979; 103:495-498

Renaud G, Foliot A, Marais J, Infanti R. Effects of clofibrate on the enzyme activity of rat liver plasma membranes. Experientia 1980; 36:281

Rennert OM. Glycoproteins in disease. Ann Clin Lab Sci 1978; 8:176-183

Reynolds HY, Atkinson JP, Newball HH, Frank MM. Receptors for immunoglobulin and complement on human alveolar macrophages. J Immunol 1975; 114:1813-1819

Roberts BE, Child JA, Cooper EH, Turner R, Stone J. Evaluation of the usefulness of serum gamma-glutamyl transpeptidase levels in the management of haematological neoplasia. Acta Haematol 1978; 59:65-72

Roberts MM, Bathgate EM, Stevenson A. Serum immunoglobulin levels in patients with breast cancer. Cancer 1975; 36:221-224

Rochman H. Tumor associated markers in clinical diagnosis. Ann Clin Lab Sci 1978; 8:167-175

Rogers AE. Variable effects of lipotrope-deficient high fat diet on chemical carcinogenesis in rats. Cancer Res 1975; 35:2469-2474

Rogers AE, Newberne PM. Dietary effects on chemical carcinogenesis in animal models for colon and liver tumors. Cancer Res 1975; 35:3427-3431

Rognum TO, Brandtzaeg P, Orjasaeter H, Fausa O. Immunohistochemistry of epithelial cell markers in normal and pathological colon mucosa. Comparison of results based on routine formalin- and cold ethanol-fixation methods. Histochemistry 1980; 67:7-21

Ronquist G, Ericsson P, Frithz G, Hugosson R. Malignant brain tumors associated with adenylate kinase in cerebrospinal fluid. Lancet 1977; 1:1284-1286

Ronquist G, Rimsten A, Westman M, Cerven E.   Serum sialyl-transferase activity in benign and malignant diseases. Acta Chim Scand 1980; 146:247-252

Rose IB.   Diagnostic studies of thyroid cancer.   J Surg Oncol 1981; 16:233-250

Rosen SE, Weintraub BD, Vaitukaitis JL, Sussman HH, Hershman JM, Muggia FM.   Placental proteins and their subunits as tumor markers.   Ann Intern Med 1975; 82:71-83

Rossen RD, Reisberg MA, Hersh EM, Gutterman JU.   The C1q binding test for soluble immune complexes: Clinical correlations obtained in patients with cancer.   J Nat Cancer Inst 1977; 58:1205-1215

Rowe DS, Hug K, Forni L, Pernis B.   Immunoglobulin D as a lymphocyte receptor.   J Exp Med 1973; 138:965-972

Rowley JD.   Chromosomal abnormalities in human leukemia. Ann Rev Genet 1980; 14:17-39

Rowley JD.   The implications of nonrandom chromosome changes for malignant transformation.   Haematol Bluttrans 1981; 26:151-155

Rubies-Prat J, Frison JC, Ras MR, Masdeu S, Moga I, Caralps A, Bacardi R.   Comparative study of X lipoprotein and gamma glutamyl transpeptidase in cholestasis and in hepatic tumors.   Rev Clin Esp 1976; 140:133-137

Ruddon RW.   ed.   Biological Markers of Neoplasia: Basic and Applied Aspects.   New York: Elsevier.   1978.   590 pp

Ruddon RW.   Role of biological markers in cancer diagnosis and treatment.   In: Biological Markers of Neoplasia: Basic and Applied Aspects.   Ruddon RW.   ed.   New York: Elsevier.   1978.   pp. 1-7

Rudman D, Chawla RK, Hendrickson LJ, Volker WR, Sophianopoulos AJ.   Isolation of a novel glycoprotein (EDC1) from the urine of a patient with acute myelocytic leukemia.   Cancer Res 1976; 36:1837-1846

Rudman D, Chawla RK, Nixon DW, Roler JH, Shah VR.   Isolation of novel glycoprotein NHC1β from urine of a patient with acute monocytic leukemia.   Cancer Res 1978; 38:602-607

Rudman D, Chawla R, Nixon DW, Vogler R, Keller JW, MacDonnel RC. Proteinuria with disseminated neoplastic disease. Cancer Res 1979; 39:699-703

Ruoslahti E, Adamson E. Alpha-fetoproteins produced by the yolk sac and the liver are glycosylated differently. Biochem Biophys Res Comm 1978; 85:1622-1630

Ruoslahti E, Pihko H. Effect of chemical modification on the immunogenicity of homologous α-fetoprotein. Ann NY Acad Sci 1975; 259:85-94

Russell DH. Clinical relevance of polyamines as biochemical markers of tumor kinetics. Clin Chem 1977; 23:22-27

Russell DH. Polyamines as markers of tumour kinetics. In: Tumour Markers: Determination and Clinical Role. Griffiths K. ed. Baltimore: University Park Press. 1978. p. 295

Russell DH, Durie BGM. Polyamines as tumor markers. Appl Methods Oncol 1979; 2:45-60

Russo AJ, Douglass HO Jr, Leveson SM, Howell JH, Holyoke ED, Harvey SR, Chu TM, Goldrosen MH. Evaluation of the micro-leukocyte adherence inhibition assay as an immunodiagnostic test for pancreatic cancer. Cancer Res 1978; 38:2023-2029

Rustin GJ. Cancer research into tumor markers. News Mirror 1980; 150:41-43

Sachdev GP, Wen G, Martin B, Kishore GS, Fox OF. Effects of dietary fat and alpha-tocopherol on gamma-glutamyltranspeptidase activity of 7,12-dimethylbenz(alpha)anthracene-induced mammary gland adenocarcinomas. Cancer Biochem Biophys 1980; 5:15-23

Sakaguchi AY, Naylor SL, Show TB, Toole JJ, McCoy M, Weinberg RA. Human c-Ki-ras2 proto-oncogene on chromosome 12. Science 1983; 219:1081-1083

Sakakibara K, Tsukada Y. Lack of correlation among gamma-glutamyltranspeptidase activity, production of alpha-fetoprotein, and transplantability in rat liver epithelial-like cell cultures. Gann 1980; 71:679-685

Sakamoto S, Kano Y, Hida K, Takaku F, Kasahara T. Enzyme markers and cellular origin of human leukemia. Nippon Ketsueki Gakkai Zasshi 1979; 42:918-932

Sala-Trepat JM, Denver J, Sargent TD, Thomas K, Sell, S. Changes in expression of albumin and α-fetoprotein genes during rat liver development and neoplasia. Biochemistry 1979; 18:2167-2178.

Salser JS, Balis ME. Fetal thymidine kinase in tumors and colonic flat mucosa of man. Nature 1976; 260:261-263

Samaan NA, Smith JP, Rutledge FN, Schultz PN. The significance of measurement of human placental lactogen, human chorionic gonadotropin, and carcinoembryonic antigen in patients with ovarian carcinoma. Am J Obstet Gynecol 1976; 126:186-189

San RH, Shimada T, Muslansky CJ, Kreiser DM, Laspia MF, Rice JM, Williams GM. Growth characteristics and enzyme activities in a survey of transformation markers in adult rat liver epithelial-like cell cultures. Cancer Res 1979; 39:4441-4448

Saravis CA, Oh SK, Pusztaszeri G, Doos W, Zamcheck N. Present status of the zinc glycinate marker (ZGM). Cancer 1978; 42:1621-1625

Sarin PS, Virmani M, Friedman B. Terminal transferase in acute lymophoblastic leukemia in gibbons. Biochim Biophys Acta 1980; 608:62-71

Sarjadi S, Daunter B, Mackay E, Mason H, Khoo SK. A multiparametric approach to the tumor markers detectable in the serum of patients with carcinoma of the ovary or uterine cervix. Gynecol Oncol 1980; 10:113-124

Sarlo K, Mortensen RF. Functional T-cell subsets required for the leukocyte adherence inhibition (LAI) measure of cellular immunity to murine sarcoma virus (MSV)-induced tumors. Proc Am Assoc Cancer Res 1982; 23:259

Savory J, Shipe JR Jr, Wills MR. Polyamines in blood-cells as cancer markers. Lancet 1979; 2:1136-1137

Sawabu N, Nakagen M, Ozaki K, Wakabayashi T, Toya D, Hattori N, Ishii M. Novel gamma-GTP isoenzyme as diagnostic tool for hepatocellular carcinoma. Ann Acad Med Singapore 1980; 9:206-209

Sawabu N, Nakagen M, Yoneda M, Makino H, Kameda S, Kobayashi K, Hattori N, Ishii M. Novel gamma-glutamyl transpeptidase isoenzyme specifically found in sera of patients with hepatocellular carcinoma. Gann 1978; 69:601-605

Sax NI. Cancer Causing Chemicals. New York: Van Nostrand Reinhold Co. 1981. 466 pp

Scalabrino G, Poso H, Holtta E. Synthesis and accumulation of polyamines in rat liver during chemical carcinogenesis. Int J Cancer 1978; 21:239-245

Scalabrino G, Terioli ME, Prerari M, Modena D, Fraschini F, Mafjorino G. Changes in the circadian rhythm of ornithine decarboxylase in rat liver during chemical hepatocarcinogenesis. J Nat Cancer Inst 1981; 66:697-702

Scheiffarth OF. T antigen and CEA: Comparison between two tumor markers in breast cancer and malignant gynecologic neoplasms. Arch Gynecol 1979; 228:659-660

Scherer E, Emmelot P. Kinetics of induction and growth of precancerous liver-cell foci, and liver tumor formation by diethylnitrosamine in the rat. Eur J Cancer 1975; 11:689-701

Scherer E, Emmelot P. Kinetics of induction and growth of enzyme-deficient islands involved in hepatocarcinogenesis. Cancer Res 1976; 36:2544-2554

Scherer E, Hoffman M, Emmelot P, Friedrich-Freksa M. Quantitative study on foci of altered liver cells induced in the rat by a single dose of diethylnitrosamine and partial hepatectomy. J Nat Cancer Inst 1972; 49:93-106

Schold SC, Wasserstrom WR, Fleisher M, Schwartz MK, Posner JB. Cerebrospinal fluid biochemical markers of central nervous system metastases. Ann Neurol 1980; 8:597-604

Schor N, Ogawa K, Lee G, Farber E. The use of the D-T diaphorase for the detection of foci of early neoplastic transformation in rat liver. Cancer Lett 1978; 6:167-171

Schulte HR, Ohde G, Schuppler J, Timmermann-Trosience I. Enhanced proliferation of putative preneoplastic cells in rat liver following treatment with tumor promotors phenobarbitol, hexachlorocyclohexane, steroid compounds, and nafenopin. Cancer Res 1981; 41:2556-2562

Schwartz MK. Enzymes in cancer--an overview. In: Biological Markers of Neoplasia: Basic and Applied Aspects. Ruddon RW, ed. New York: Elsevier. 1978. pp. 503-515

Schwartz MK. Biochemical and immunochemical markers associated with cancer. Clin Bull 1976; 6:62-68

Schwartz MK. Laboratory aids to diagnosis--enzymes. Cancer 1976; 37:542-548

Schwartz MK. Tumor markers, enzymes and hormonal markers. Clin Gastroenterol 1976; 5:653-663

Schwartz TW. Pancreatic-polypeptide (PP) and endocrine tumours of the pancreas. Scand J Gastroenterol Suppl 1979; 14:93-100

Seidenfeld J, Marton LJ. Biochemical markers of central nervous system tumors in cerebrospinal fluid. Ann Clin Lab Sci 1978; 8:459-466

Seidenfeld J, Marton LJ. Biochemical markers of central nervous system tumors measured in cerebrospinal fluid and their potential use in diagnosis and patient management: A review. J Nat Cancer Inst 1979; 63:919-931

Seiler N, Graham A, Bortholeyns J. Enhanced urinary excretion of N^1-acetylspermidine and the presence of tumors. Cancer Res 1981; 41:1572-1573

Sell S. Radioimmunoassay of rat α-fetoprotein. Cancer Res 1973; 33:1010-1015

Sell S. Studies on rabbit-lymphocytes in vitro. XIX. Kinetics of reversible antiallotypic stimulation and restimulation of blast transformation. Cell Immunol 1974; 12:119-126

Sell S. Distribution of α-fetoprotein- and albumin-containing cells in the livers of Fischer rats fed four cycles of N-2-fluorenylacetamide. Cancer Res 1978; 38: 3107-3113

Sell S. Alpha fetoprotein. In: Cancer Markers: Diagnostic and Developmental Significance. Sell S. ed. Clifton NJ: Humana Press. 1980. pp. 249-294

Sell S. ed. Cancer Markers: Diagnostic and Developmental Significance. Clifton NJ: Humana Press. 1980. 541 pp

Sell S, Becker FF. Guest Editorial: Alpha fetoprotein. J Nat Cancer Inst 1978; 60:19-26

Sell S, Becker FF, Lombardi B, Shinozuka H, Reddy J. Alpha-fetoprotein production by normal and abnormal liver cells. II. Differences in the sequence of morphologic events and kinetics of elevation of serum AFP during chemical induction of lung cancer. In: Lehman FG. ed. Carcinoembryonic Proteins, Vol. 1. New York: Elsevier-North Holland Press, 1979, pp. 129-136

Sell S, Leffert HL. An evaluation of cellular lineages in the pathogenesis of experimental hepatocellular carcinoma. Hepatology 1982; 2:77-86

Sell S, Stillman D, Gochman N. Serum alpha-fetoprotein: A prognostic indicator of liver cell necrosis and regeneration following experimental injury by galactosamine in rats. Am J Clin Pathol 1976; 66:847-883

Sell S, Stillman D, Michaelson M, Alaimo J, von Essen C. Prevention of pulmonary metastasis by irradiation of the lung: A model system employing a transplantable hepatoma and alpha$_1$ fetoprotein as an index of tumor growth. Radiat Res 1977; 69:54-64

Sell S, Wahren B. Human Cancer Markers. Clifton NJ: Humana Press. 1982. 428 pp

Sell S, Wepsic HT, Nickel R, Nichols M. Rat alpha feto-protein. IV. Effects of growth and surgical removal of Morris hepatoma 7777 on the serum α_1F concentration of buffalo rats. J Nat Cancer Inst 1974; 52:133-137

Sella A, Wysenbeek AJ, Yeshurun D. Adenocarcinoma of the lung secreting alkaline phosphatase. Respiration 1979; 38:180-183

Sells MA, Katyal SL, Sell S, Shinozuka H, Lombardi B. Induction of foci of altered, gamma-glutamyltranspepti-dase-positive hepatocytes in carcinogen-treated rats fed a choline-deficient diet. Br J Cancer 1979; 40:274-283

Selvaraj P, Balasubramanian KA, Hill PG. Isolation of gamma-glutamyl transpeptidase from human primary hepatoma and comparison of its kinetic and catalytic properties with the enzyme from normal adult and fetal liver. Enzyme 1981; 26:57-63

Seppala M, Wahlstrom T, Bohn H. Circulating levels and tissue localization of placental protein (PP5) in pregnancy and trophoblastic disease: Absence of PP5 expression in the malignant trophoblast. Int J Cancer 1979; 24:6-10

Sessa A, Desiderio MA, Baizini M, Perin A. Diamine oxidase activity in regenerating rat liver and in 4-dimethylaminobenzene-induced and Yoshida AH 130 hepatomas. Cancer Res 1981; 41:1929-1934

Sethi JK, Hirshaut Y. Characterization of human sarcoma antigen S3. Br J Cancer 1981; 43:261-166

Sharma RK, Ahrens H, Shanker G, Moore RE. Regulation of a novel autophosphorylating protein kinase by adrenocortical carcinoma: A review. Cell Mol Biol 1980; 26:65-73

Sharma RN, Gurtoo HL, Farber E, Murray RK, Cameron RG. Effects of hepatocarcinogens and hepatocarcinogenesis on the activity of rat liver microsomal epoxide hydrolase and observations on the electrophoretic behavior of this enzyme. Cancer Res 1981; 41:3311-3319

Shatton JB, Harshida S, Williams A, Morris HP, Weinhouse S. Activities and properties of inorganic pyrophosphatase in normal tissues and hepatic tumors of the rat. Cancer Res 1981; 41:1866-1872

Sheid B, Lu T, Nelson JH Jr. Transfer RNA methylase activity in benign human ovarian neoplasms. Cancer Res 1974; 34:2416-2418

Sheid B, Lu T, Pedrinan L, Nelson JH Jr. Plasma ribonuclease. A marker for the detection of ovarian cancer. Cancer 1977; 38:2204-2208

Sheinina LI, Kutivadye DA. ATPase and 5'-nucleotidase in human breast and stomach tumors. Arch Pathol 1980; 42: 35-38

Shih C, Shilo BZ, Goldfarb MP, Dannenberg A, Weinberg RA. Passage of phenotypes of chemically transformed cells via transfection of DNA and chromatin. Proc Nat Acad Sci USA 1981; 76:5714-5718

Shimada T, San RH, Williams GM. Quantitative markers for transformation of cultured rat liver epithelial cells. Ann NY Acad Sci 1980; 349:397-398

Shimizu M, Fujimura S. Studies on the abnormal excretion of pyrimidine nucleosides in the urine of Yoshida ascites sarcoma-bearing rats. Increased excretion of deoxycytidine, pseudouridine and cytidine. Biochim Biophys Acta 1978; 517:277-286

Shinozuka H, Katyal SL, Lombardi B. Azaserine carcinogenesis: Organ susceptibility change in rats fed a diet devoid of choline. Int J Cancer 1978a; 22:36-39

Shinozuka H, Lombardi B, Sell S, Iammarino RM. Enhancement of ethionine liver carcinogenesis in rats fed a choline devoid diet. J Nat Cancer Inst 1978b; 61:813-817

Shinozuka H, Sells MA, Katyal SL. Effects of choline-devoid diet on the emergence of alpha-glutamyltranspeptidase-positive foci in the liver of carcinogen-treated rats. Cancer Res 1979; 39:2515-2521

Shipe JR, Savory J, Wills MR, Rowley R, Looney WB, Hopkins HA. Erythrocyte polyamine levels in rats with H4IIE hepatomas before and after radiation treatment. Res Commun Chem Pathol Pharmacol 1980; 28:329-342

Shively JE, Toss CW. Carcinoembryonic antigen. In: Cancer Markers: Diagnostic and Developmental Significance. Sell S. ed. Clifton NJ: Humana Press. 1980. pp. 295-314

Shuttleworth E, Allen N. CSF beta-glucuronidase assay in the diagnosis of neoplastic meningitis. Arch Neurol 1980; 37:684-697

Silva OM, Becker KL. Calcitonin as a marker for cancer. In: Biological Markers of Neoplasia: Basic and Applied Aspects. Ruddon RW. ed. New York: Elsevier. 1978. pp. 295-310

Silver HK, Karim KA, Salinas FA. Relationship of total serum sialic acid to sialylglycoprotein acute-phase reactants in malignant melanoma. Br J Cancer 1980; 41:745-750

Silver HKB, Karim KA, Gray MJ, Salinas FA. High performance liquid chromatography quantitation of N-acetylneuraminic

acid in malignant melanoma and breast carcinoma.
J Chromatogr 1981; 224:381-388

Silverman LM, Dermer AB, Tokes ZA. Electrophoretic patterns
for serum glycoproteins reflect the presence of human
breast cancer. Clin Chem 1977; 23:2055-2058

Simiskova M, Dolezalova V, Nemecek R. Correlation of
deoxycytidylate deaminase activity with cell proliferation
during hepatocarcinogenesis and tumor growth in transplantable rat hepatomas. Folia Biol (Prague) 1980; 26:
194-203

Singh N, Clausen J. Different tissue responses of mixed
function oxidases and detoxifying enzymes to aflatoxin B_1
administration in the rat. Br J Exp Pathol 1980; 61:611-
616

Sizaret P, Esteve J. Relative potencies of four CEA
preparations by three commercial radioimmunoassay kits.
J Immunol Methods 1980; 34:79-92

Sizemore GW, Carney JA, Heath H. Epidemiology of medullary
carcinoma of the thyroid gland: A 5-year experience
(1971-1976). Surg Clin N Am 1977; 57:633-645

Sjögren HO, Hellström I, Bansal SC, Hellström KE.
Suggestive evidence that the "blocking antibodies" of
tumour-bearing individuals may be antigen-antibody
complexes. Proc Nat Acad Sci USA 1971; 68:1372-1375

Sjögren HO, Hellström I, Bansal SC, Warner GA,
Hellström KE. Elution of blocking factors from human
tumours capable of abrogating tumour-cell destruction
by specifically immune lymphocytes. Int J Cancer 1972;
9:274-283

Sjögren HO, Steele G Jr. The immunology of large bowel
carcinoma in a rat model. Cancer 1975; 36:2469-2471

Sloane JP, Ormerod MG, Neville AM. Potential pathological
application of immunocytochemical methods to the detection
of micrometastases. Cancer Res 1980; 40:3079-3082

Smuckler EA, Kaplitz M, Sell S. α-Fetoprotein responses
following phenobarbital stimulation of rat liver. In:
Oncodevelopmental Gene Expression. Fishman WH, Sell S.
eds. New York: Academic Press. 1975. pp. 247-251

Snodgrass DR, McLemore TL, Teague RB, Wray NP, Busbee DL. Aryl hydrocarbon hydroxylase activity in pulmonary macrophages and blood lymphocytes. Asbestos-exposed cigarette smokers with and without lung cancer. Chest 1981; 80: 42-44

Snyder PJ, Johnson J, Muzyka R. Abnormal secretion of glycoprotein alpha-subunit and follicle-stimulating hormone (FSH) beta-subunit in men with pituitary adenomas and FSH hypersecretion. J Clin Endocrinol Metab 1980; 51:579-584

Solanki RL, Ramdeo IN, Sachdev KN. Serum protein bound fucose in diagnosis of breast malignancy. Indian J Med Res 1978; 67:786-791

Soloff MS, Swartz SK, Pearlmutter SF, Kithier K. Binding of 17β-estradiol by variants of α-fetoprotein in rat amniotic fluid. Biochim Biophys Acta 1976; 427:644-651

Soloff MS, Creange JE, Potts GO. Unique estrogen-binding properties of rat pregnancy plasma. Endocrinol 1971; 88:427-432

Solomon A. Monoclonal immunoglobulins as biomarkers of cancer. In: Cancer Markers. Diagnostic and Developmental Significance. Sell S. ed. Clifton NJ: Humana Press. 1980. pp. 57-87

Solt D, Farber E. A new principle for the sequential analysis of chemical carcinogenesis including a quantitative assay for initiation in liver. Nature 1976; 263:701-703

Solt D, Medline A, Farber E. Rapid emergence of carcinogen-induced hyperplastic lesions in a new model for the sequential analysis of liver carcinogenesis. Am J Pathol 1977; 88:595-618

Solt D. Localization of gamma-glutamyl transpeptidase in hamster buccal pouch epithelium treated with 7,12-dimethylbenz(a)anthracene. J Nat Cancer Inst 1981; 67: 193-200

Speer J, Gehrke CW, Kuo KC, Waalkes TP, Borek E. tRNA breakdown products as markers for cancer. Cancer 1979; 44:2120-2123

Springer GF, Murthy SM, Desai PR, Fry WA, Tegtmeyer H, Scanlon EF. Patients' immune response to breast and lung carcinoma-associated Thomsen-Friedenreich (T) specificity. Klin. Wochenschr. 1982; 60:121-131

Srivastava BIS, Khan SA, Minowada J. Terminal deoxynucleotidyl transferase activity and blast cell characteristics in adult human leukemias. Leuk Res 1980; 4:209-215

Staab HJ, Anderer FA, Hiesche K, Wehrle E, Rodatz W. Is serum beta-2-microglobulin a tumor marker in gastrointestinal cancer? Clin Chim Acta 1980; 106:309-317

Stanhope CR, Smith JP, Britton JC, Crosley PK. Serial determination of marker substances in ovarian cancer. Gynecol Oncol 1979; 8:284-287

Stass SA, Shumacher HR, Keneklin TP, Bollum FJ. Terminal deoxynucleotidyl transferase immunofluorescence of bone marrow smears. Experience in 156 cases. Am J Clin Pathol 1979; 72:889-903

Statland BE. The challenge of cancer testing. Research update: Tumor markers. Diagn Med 1981; June special issue, pp. 12-38

Statland BE. Guest Editorial. Diagn Med 1981; 4:1

Steele GJ, Sjögren HO. Cross-reacting tumor-associated antigen(s) among chemically induced rat colon carcinomas. Cancer Res 1974; 34:1801-1807

Stevans RH, Cole CA, Cheng HF. Identification of a common oncofetal protein in X-ray and chemically induced rat gastrointestinal tumours. Br J Cancer 1981; 43:817-825

Stewart BW. Generation and persistence of carcinogen-induced repair intermediates in rat liver DNA in vivo. Cancer Res 1981; 41:3238-3243

Stimson WH. Protein markers in disease (2). Pregnancy-associated α_2-glycoprotein and cancer. J R Coll Surg Edinb 1978; 23:253-259

Stocco DM, Hutson JC. Characteristics of mitochondria isolated by rate zonal centrifugation from normal liver and Novikoff hepatomas. Cancer Res 1980; 40:1486-1492

Stolbach LL, Krant MJ, Fishman WH. Ectopic production of an alkaline phosphatase isozyme in patients with cancer. New Engl J Med 1969; 281:757-762

Stora C, Aussel C, Lafaurie M, Kreb B, Ayraud N. On the synthesis of alfa-fetoprotein during liver carcinogenesis by N-2-fluorenylacetamide and its relationships with intracellular localization of the carcinogen. Oncology 1981; 38:43-46

Strong DD, Herschman HR. Identification and character-ization of a brain-specific antigen enriched in neonatal brain. II. Antigenic stability, species cross-reactivity and tumor cell association. Brain Res 1980; 184:271-282

Sugar J, Szentirmay Z, Kralovansky J. Pathological features of N-methyl-N'-nitro-N-nitrosoguanidine induced neoplastic and preneoplastic lesions of rat stomach. IARC Sci Publ 1980; 31:667-675

Suzuki H. Clinical significance of appearance of serum gamma-glutamyl transpeptidase isozyme. Gastroenterol Jpn 1981; 16:122-128

Szymanovicz A, Joubert PM, Barbe A. An automatic technique for the routine fractionation of the urinary hydroxypro-line containing peptides. Clin Chim Acta 1980; 199: 155-164

Szymendera JJ, Zborzil J, Sikorowa L, Kaminska JA, Gadek A. Value of five tumor markers (AFP, CEA, hCG, hPL, and SP_1) in diagnosis and staging of testicular germ cell tumors. Oncology 1981; 38:222-229

Tabin CJ, Bradley SM, Bargmann CI, Weinberg RA, Papageorge AG, Scolnick EM, Dhar R, Lowy DR, Chang EH. Mechanism of activation of a human oncogene. Nature 1982; 300:143-149

Takahashi S, Katyal SL, Lombardi B, Shinozuka H. Induction of foci of altered hepatocytes by a single injection of azaserine to rats. Cancer Lett 1979; 7:265-272

Takami H, Nishioka K. Raised polyamines in erythrocytes from melanoma-bearing mice and patients with solid tumor. Br J Cancer 1980; 41:751-756

Takami H, Romsdahl MM, Nishioka K. Polyamines in blood-cells as cancer markers. Lancet 1979; 2:912

Takeuchi J, Handa H, Suda K, Aso T. In vitro secretion of follicle-stimulating hormone by pituitary chromophobe adenomas. Surg Neurol 1980; 14:303-309

Takeuchi T, Mara M, Sasake R, Matsushima T, Sugimura T. Comparative studies on electrophoretic mobility and immunogenicity of pancreatic and parotid amylases of rat. Biochem Biophys Acta 1975; 403:456-460

Takeuchi T, Nakayasu M, Hirohashi S, Kameya T, Kaneko M, Yokomore K, Tsuchida Y. Human endodermal sinus tumor in nude mice and its markers for diagnosis and management. J Clin Pathol 1979; 32:693-699

Tamano S, Tsuda H, Tatematsu M, Hasegawa R, Imaida K, Ito N. Induction of γ-glutamyl transpeptidase positive foci in rat liver by pyrolysis products of amino acids. Gann 1981; 72:747-753

Tamura S, Matsumoto Y. Comparative studies on postnatal development of liver beta-glucuronidase activity between Gunn rats and Wistar rats. J Toxicol Sci 1980; 5:331-338

Taniguchi N. Purification and some properties of γ-glutamyl transpeptidase from azo dye-induced hepatoma. J Biochem Tokyo 1974; 75:473-480

Taniguchi N, Saito K, Takakuwa E. γ-Glutamyltransferase from azo dye induced hepatoma and fetal rat liver: Similarities in their kinetic and imunological properties. Biochim Biophys Acta 1975; 391:265-271

Taniguchi N, Tsukada Y, Mukuo K, Hirai H. Effect of hepatocarcinogenic azo dyes on glutathione and related enzymes in rat liver. Gann 1974; 65:381-387

Tarro G. Analysis and description of procedures used in the study of the relationship of herpes simplex virus "non-virion" antigens to certain cancers. IARC Sci Publ 1975; 11:191-297

Tartter PI, Slater G, Gelernt I, Aupes AH. Screening for liver metastases from colorectal cancer with carcinoembryonic antigen and alkaline phosphatase. Ann Surg 1981; 193:357-360

Tatarinov YS. Obnaruzhenie embriospetificheskogo alpha-globulina v syvorotke krovi bol'nogo pervichnym rakom pecheni. Vop Med Khim 1964; 10:90-91

Tatarinov YS. Trophoblast-specific β_2-glycoprotein as a marker for pregnancy and malignancies. Gynecol Obstet Invest 1978; 9:65-97

Tataryn DN, MacFarlane JK, Thomson DM. Leukocyte adherence inhibition for detecting specific tumor immunity in early pancreatic cancer. Lancet 1978; 5:1020-1022

Tate SS, Thompson GA, Meister A. Recent studies on γ-glutamyltranspeptidase. In: Glutathione: Metabolism and Function. Arias IM, Jakoby WB. eds. New York: Raven Press. 1976. pp. 45-61

Tatematsu M, Nakanishi K, Murasaki G, Miyata Y, Hirose M, Ito N. Enhancing effect of inducers of liver microsomal enzymes on induction of hyperplastic liver nodules by N-2-fluorenylacetamide in rats. J Nat Cancer Inst 1979; 63: 1411-1416

Tatematsu M, Shirai T, Tsuda H, Miyata Y, Shinohara Y, Ito N. Rapid production of hyperplastic liver nodules in rats treated with carcinogenic chemicals: A new approach for an in vivo short-term screening test for hepatocarcinogens. Gann 1977; 68:499-507

Taylor CR, Klezdik G. Immunohistologic techniques in surgical pathology--a spectrum of "new" special stains. Human Pathol 1981; 12:590-596

Thakore KN, Nigam SK, Karnik AB, Lakkad BC, Bhatt DK, Babu KA, Kashyap SK, Chatterjee SK. Early changes in serum protein and liver LDH isoenzymes in mice exposed to technical grade hexachlorocyclohexane (BHC) and their possible relationship to liver tumours. Toxicology 1981; 19:31-37

Theofilopoulos AN, Andrews BS, Urist MM, Morton DL, Dixon FJ. The nature of immune complexes in human cancer sera. J Immunol 1977; 119:657-663

Thomale J, Nass G. Elevated urinary excretion of RNA catabolites as an early signal of tumor development in mice. Cancer Lett 1982; 15:149-159

Thompson MB, Dent JG, Graichen ME, Neptun DA, Scortichini BH, Popp JA. Effects of α-naphthylisothiocyanate, lithocholic acid and selected hepatocarcinogens on epoxide hydrolase, DT-diaphorase and serum indicators of cholestasis. Toxicologist 1982; 2:101

Thompson SW, Vladislava SR. Some thoughts on attempts to correlate the occurrence of neoplastic and non-neoplastic spontaneous diseases in laboratory animals. Toxicol Pathol 1981; 9:1-18

Thomson DM. Demonstration of tube leukocyte adherence inhibition assay with coded samples of blood. Cancer Res 1979; 39:627-629

Thomson DM, Tataryn DN, O'Connor R, Ranch J, Friedlander P, Gold P, Shuster J. Evidence for the expression of human tumor-specific antigens associated with B12-microglobulin in human cancer and in some colon adenomas and benign breast lesions. Cancer Res 1979; 39:604-611

Thomson DPM. ed. Assessment of Immune Status by the Leukocyte Adherence Inhibition Test. New York: Academic Press. 1982. 380 pp

Thung SN, Gerber MA. Enzyme pattern and marker antigens in nodular "regenerative" hyperplasia of the liver. Cancer 1981; 47:1796-1799

Thynne GS. Plasma carcinoembryonic antigen and erythrocyte sedimentation rate in patients with colorectal carcinoma. Med J Aust 1979; 1:592-593

Thynne GS, Greening WP. A correlation of erythrocyte sedimentation and plasma carcinoembryonic antigen in fibrocystic disease and carcinoma of the breast. Clin Oncol 1980; 6:317-321

Tietz NW. Fundamentals of Clinical Chemistry. Philadelphia: W. B. Saunders Co. 1976a. pp. 652-657

Tietz NW. Fundamentals of Clinical Chemistry. Philadelphia: W. B. Saunders Co. 1976b. pp. 602-604

Tizard IR. ed. An Introduction to Veterinary Immunology. Philadelphia: W. B. Saunders Co. 1977. pp. 335-343

Tomatis L. The predictive value of rodent carcinogenicity tests in the evaluation of human risks. Ann Rev Pharmacol Toxicol 1979; 19:511-530

Tormey DC, Coates AS, Whitehead RP. Circulating tumor markers. In: Endocrinological Cancer, Vol. 2. Rose DP. ed. Boca Raton FL: CRC Press. 1979. pp. 125-148

Tormey DC, Waalkes TP. Biochemical markers in cancer of the breast. Recent Results Cancer Res 1976; 57:78-94

Torti FM, Carter DK. The chemotherapy of prostatic adeno-carcinoma. Ann Intern Med 1980; 92:681-689

Toshitsugu O, Hiroshi S, Yasuo E. Clinico-chemical biochem-ical diagnosis of hepatomas. Gann to Kagaku Ryoko 1978; 5:381-387

Tottori K. Diagnostic and follow-up studies on carcinofetal proteins in the sera of gynecological malignancies. Acta Obstet Gynecol Jpn 1979; 31:2193-2202

Trump BF, Heatfield BM, Phelps PC, Sanefuji H, Shamsuddin AK. Cell surface changes in preneoplastic and neoplastic epithelium. Scanning Electron Microsc 1980; 3:43-60

Tsou KC, Lo KW. Serum 5'-nucleotide phosphodiesterase isozyme-V test for human liver cancer. Cancer 1980; 45:209-213

Tsou KC, Lo KW, Herberman RB, Schutt AJ. Detection of liver metastases with 5'-nucleotide phosphodiesterase isozyme-V in gastrointestinal cancer patients. Oncology 1980; 37: 381-385

Tsuchida S, Hoshino K, Sato T, Ito N, Sato K. Purification of gamma-glutamyltransferase from rat hepatomas and hyper-plastic hepatic nodules, and comparison with the enzyme from rat kidney. Cancer Res 1979; 39:4200-4205

Tsuda H, Farber E. Resistant hepatocytes as early changes in liver induced by polycyclic aromatic hydrocarbons. Int J Cancer 1980; 25:137-139

Tsuda H, Lee G, Farber E. Induction of resistant hepato-cytes as a new principle for a possible short-term in vivo test for carcinogens. Cancer Res 1980; 40:1157-1164

Twardzik DR, Todaro GJ, Marquardt H, Reynolds FH Jr, Stephenson JR. Transformation induced by Abelson murine leukemia virus involves production of a polypeptide growth factor. Science 1982; 216:894-897

Tyndall RL, Clapp NK, Davidson KA, Colyer SP, Burtis CA. Effects of carcinogenic and non-carcinogenic chemicals on

plasma esterases in BALB/c mice. Chem Biol Interact 1978;
23:159-169

Uchida T, Miyata H, Shikata T. Human hepatocellular carcinoma and putative precancerous disorders: Their enzyme
histochemical study. Arch Pathol Lab Med 1981; 105:
180-186

Uchijima Y, Kurokawa J, Akutsu M, Okada K, Komase M.
Clinical studies on testicular tumors: Serum markers and
the clinical course of the tumor. J Saitama Med School
1979; 6:365-376

Uehara N, Shirakawa S, Uchino H, Saeki Y, Nozaki M.
Elevated polyamine levels in erythrocytes of SLC:ICR mice
inoculated with Ehrlich ascites carcinoma cells. Life Sci
1980; 26:461-467

Unanue ER, Grey HM, Rabellino Z, Campbell P, Schmitke J.
Immunoglobulins on the surface of lymphocytes. II. The
bone marrow as the main source of lymphocytes with
detectable surface-bound immunoglobulin. J Exp Med
1971; 133:1188-1198

Ungerleider RS. Working conference on neuroblastoma
treatment trials. Cancer Treat Rep 1981; 65:719-723

Uotila P. Effects of single and repeated cigarette smoke
exposures on the activities of aryl hydrocarbon hydroxylase, epoxide hydratase and UDP glucuronosyl transferase
in rat lung, kidney and small intestinal mucosa. Res
Commun Chem Pathol Pharmacol 1977; 17:101-114

USDHEW. Oncology Overview: Selected Abstracts on
Pancreatic Carcinogenesis. 1980

U.S. Public Health Service. Second annual report on
carcinogens: December 1981, NTP Publ. No. 81-43.
Washington DC: U.S. Government Printing Office

U.S. Public Health Service. Healthy people: The Surgeon
General's report on health promotion and disease preven-
tion, DHEW (PHS) Publ. No. 79-55071. Washington DC: U.S.
Government Printing Office. 1979

U.S. Public Health Service. Surveillance epidemiology, end
results. Incidence and mortality data: 1973-77. NCI
Monograph 57. U.S. Dept. of Health and Human Resources

Vaitukaitis JL, Braunstein GC, Ross GT. A radioimmune assay which specifically measures human chorionic gonadotropin in the presence of human luteinizing hormone. Am J Obstet Gynecol 1972; 113:751-758

Van Wijk R, Louwers HA, Bisschop A. The induction of ornithine decarboxylase and DNA synthesis in rat hepatocytes after a single administration of diethylnitrosamine. Carcinogenesis 1981; 2:27-31

Veltri RW, Mengoli HF, Maxim PE, Westfall S, Gopo JM, Hauang CW, Sprinkle PM. Isolation and identification of human lung tumor-associated antigens. Cancer Res 1977; 37:1313-1322

Vezzoni P, Campagnari F, DiFronzo G, Clerici L. Terminal deoxynucleotidyl transferase in human lymphomas: Possible existence of forms with high and low molecular weights. Br J Cancer 1981; 43:312-319

Vihko P, Kostama A, Janne O. Rapid radioimmunoassay for prostate-specific acid phosphatase in human serum. Clin Chem 1980; 26:1544-1547

Viot M, Joulin C, Cambon P, Krebs BP. The value of serum alkaline phosphatase alpha 1 isoenzyme in the diagnosis of liver metastases. Preliminary results. Biomed Express (Paris) 1979; 31:74-77

Vladutin AO, Brason FW, Adler RH. Differential diagnosis of pleural effusions: Clinical usefulness of cell marker quantitation. Chest 1981; 79:297-301

Volm VM, Wayss K, Wesch H, Zimmerer J. Korrelation Zwischen der Kupfer und Caeruloplasmin Konzentration im Plasma und dem ^{3}H-thymidin-Einbau de Walker-Karzinosarkoms. Arch Geschwulstforsch 1972; 40:248-258

Waalkes TP, Tormey DC. Biologic markers and breast cancer. Semin Oncol 1978; 5:434-444

Waalkes TP, Gehrke CW, Tormey DC, Woo KB, Kuo KC, Synder J, Hansen H. Biologic markers in breast carcinoma. IV. Serum fucose-protein ratio. Comparisons with carcinoembryonic antigen and human chorionic gonadotrophin. Cancer 1978; 41:1871-1882

Waalkes TP, Gehrke CW, Zumwalt RW, Chang SY, Lakings DB, Tormey DC, Ahman DL, Moertel CG. The urinary excretion of nucleosides of ribonucleic acid by patients with advanced cancer. Cancer 1975; 36:390-398

Waalkes TP, Mrochek JE, Dinsmore SR, Tormey DC. Serum protein-bound carbohydrates for following the course of disease in patients with metastatic breast carcinoma. J Nat Cancer Inst 1978; 61:703-707

Wahren B, Holmgren PA, Stigbrand T. Placental alkaline phosphatase, alphafetoprotein and carcinoembryonic antigen in testicular tumors. Tissue typing by means of cytologic smears. Int J Cancer 1979; 24:749-753

Wainfan E, Brody H, Balis ME. A sensitive assay for carcinogen-induced early changes in tRNA methyltransferase activity. Proc Am Assoc Cancer Res 1979; 20:65

Wainfan E, Brody H, Balis ME. Reversible changes in rat liver tRNA methyltransferase activities induced by carbon tetrachloride. Proc Am Assoc Cancer Res 1981; 22:79

Wainfan E, Tscherne JS, Maschio FA, Balis ME. Time dependence of ethionine-induced changes in rat liver transfer RNA methylation. Cancer Res 1977; 37:865-869

Waldman SR, Yonemoto RH. The use of cryopreserved lymphocytes in the leukocyte adherence inhibition assay. I. Evaluation of specificity of responses in cancer patients. Int J Cancer 1978; 21:542-551

Warnock M, Press M, Chung A. Further observations on cytoplasmic hyaline in the lung. Human Pathol 1980; 11:59

Warren L. The thiobarbituric acid assay of sialic acids. J Biol Chem 1959; 234:1971-1975

Warwas M, Narczeuskz B, Dobryszycka W. Blood serum peptidases in patients with ovarian carcinoma treated with Ledakrin. Arch Immunol Ther Exp 1977; 25:235-242

Wasserstrom WR, Schwartz MK, Fleisher M, Posner JB. Cerebrospinal fluid biochemical markers in central nervous system tumors: A review. Ann Clin Lab Sci 1981; 11: 239-251

Watabe H. Early appearance of embryonic α-globulin in rat serum during carcinogenesis with 4-methyl aminobenzene. Cancer Res 1971; 31:1192-1194

Watabe H. Purification and chemical characterization of α-fetoprotein from rat and mouse. Int J Cancer 1974; 13: 377–388

Watabe H, Nishi S, Hirai H. Further investigation on AFP in rats subjected to chemical hepatocarcinogenesis. Tumor Res 1973; 8:71–74

Watanabe H, Hakamori SI. Status of blood group carbohydrate chains in ontogenesis and in oncogenesis. J Exp Med 1976; 144:645–653

Watanabe K, Williams GM. Enhancement of rat hepatocellular altered foci by the liver tumor promoter phenobarbital: Evidence that the foci are precursors of neoplasms and that the promoter acts on carcinogen-induced lesions. J Nat Cancer Inst 1978; 61:1311–1314

Watring WG, Edinger DD Jr, Anderson B. Screening and diagnosis in ovarian cancer. Clin Obstet Gynecol 1979; 22:745–757

Watson RA, Tang DB. The predictive value of prostatic acid phosphatase as a screening test for prostatic cancer. New Engl J Med 1980; 303:494–499

Waxman S, Liu CK, Schmied R. Abnormal glycoproteins and glycosyltransferases in human hepatoma. Ann NY Acad Sci 1980; 349:411–412

Webber MM, Buffkin DC, Juillard GJ, Schwabe AD, Verma RC, Bennet LR. Ornithine metabolism in normal subjects and patients with cancer. J Nucl Med 1980; 21:1194–1196

Weickmann JL, Glitz DG. Human ribonucleases: Quantitation of pancreatic-like enzymes in serum, urine, and organ preparations. J Biol Chem 1982; 257:8705–8710

Weinberg RA. Fewer and fewer oncogenes. Cell 1982; 30:3–4

Weisburger JH, Williams GM. Carcinogen testing: Current problems and new approaches. Science 1981; 214:401–407

Weiser MM, Wilson JR. Serum levels of glycosyltransferases and related glycoproteins as indicators of cancer: Biological and clinical implications. CRC Crit Rev Clin Lab Sci 1981; 14:189–239

Weiser MM, Podolsky DK, Isselbacher KJ. Cancer-associated isoenzyme of serum galactosyltransferase. Proc Nat Acad Sci USA 1976; 73:1319-1322

Weissman B, Bromberg PA, Gutman AM. The purine bases of human urine. II. Semiquantitative estimation and isotope incorporation. J Biol Chem 1957; 224:423-434

Wepsic HT, Tracey RS, Seoo S, Harris S, Ribi E, Morris H. BCG cell wall immunotherapy of intramuscular and meta-static Morris rat hepatoma. Cancer Res 1978; 38:1217-1222

Westerbrink K, Havsteen B. High-resolution 2-dimensional electrophoresis of protein-fractions from samples of normal human-tissue and of tumors: Computer search for novel tumor-markers. Hoppe-Seyler's Z Physiol Chem 1982; 363:908

Whitehead JS, Fearney FJ, Kim YS. Glycosyltransferase and glycosidase activities in cultured human fetal and colonic adenocarcinoma cell lines. Cancer Res 1979; 39:1259-1263

Williams GM. Pathogenesis of rat liver cancer caused by chemical carcinogens. Biochim Biophys Acta 1980; 605:167-189

Williams GM, Hirota N, Rice JM. The resistance of sponta-neous mouse hepatocellular neoplasms to iron accumulation during rapid iron loading by parenteral administration and their transplantability. Am J Pathol 1979; 94:65-74

Williams GM, Ohmori T, Katayama S, Rice JM. Alteration by phenobarbital of membrane-associated enzymes including gamma glutamyltranspeptidase in mouse liver neoplasms. Carcinogenesis 1980; 1:813-818

Williams GM, Watanabe K. Quantitative kinetics of development of N-2-fluorenylacetamide-induced, altered (hyperplastic) hepatocellular foci resistant to iron accumulation and of their reversion or persistance following removal of carcinogen. J Nat Cancer Inst 1978; 61:113-121

Wilson PD, Hodges GM. Focal distribution of surface marker enzymes after long-term culture of adult rat bladder epithelium and methylnitrosourea (MNU)-induced bladder tumors. J Histochem Cytochem 1979; 27:1236-1246

Winicov I. Liver and kidney nuclear RNA synthesis and modifications in dimethylnitrosamine-treated rats. Biochim Biophys Acta 1981; 654:31-41

Wise KS, Muller E. γ-Glutamyl transpeptidase in human nephroblastoma grown in nude mice. Speciala 1976; 15:294-296

Wolberg WH, Morin J. Thymidylate synthetase activity and fluorouracil sensitivity of human colonic cancer and normal mucosal tissue preparations. Cancer 1981; 47:1313-1317

Wolf PL, Ray G, Kaplan H. Evaluation of copper oxidase (ceruloplasmin) and related tests in Hodgkin's disease. Clin Biochem 1979; 12:202-204

Woods JC, Spriggs AI, Harris H, McGee JO. A new marker for human cancer cells. 3. Immunocytochemical detection of malignant cells in serous fluids with the Ca antibody. Lancet 1982; 8297:512-514

Wuhan Medical College, Department of Pathophysiology, Wuhan, China. Possibility of immunodiagnosis in ovarian cancer. Gynecol Obstet Invest 1978; 9:98-108

Ying TS, Sarma DSR, Farber E. The sequential analysis of liver cell necrosis. Inhibition of diethylnitrosamine- and dimethylnitrosamine-induced acute liver cell death by posttreatment with diethyldithiocarbamate. Am J Pathol 1980; 99:159-174

Ying TS, Sarma DSR, Farber E. Role of acute hepatic necrosis in the induction of early steps in liver carcinogenesis by diethylnitrosamine. Cancer Res 1981; 41:2096-2102

Ylikorkala O, Kauppila A, Rajala T. Pituitary gonodatrophins and prolactin in patients with endometrial cancer, fibroids or ovarian tumors. Br J Obstet Gynaecol 1979; 86:901-904

Yogeeswaran G. Surface glycolipid and glycoprotein antigens. In: Cancer Markers: Diagnostic and Developmental Significance. Sell S. ed. Clifton NJ: Humana Press. 1980. pp. 371-401

Yokota T, Katahira S, Konno K, Minami K. Attempts to seek oncofetal antigens on rat liver cells transformed in vitro by chemical carcinogens. Fukushima J Med Sci 1979; 26:11-29

Zubler RH, Lange G, Lambert PH, Meischer PA. Detection of immune complexes in unheated sera by modified ^{125}I-C1q binding test. Effect on the binding of C1q by immune complexes and application of the test to systemic lupus erythematosus. J Immunol 1976; 116:232-235

Zweig MH, Van Steirteghem AC. Assessment of radioimmunoassay of serum creatine kinase BB (CK-BB) as a tumor marker: Studies in patients with various cancers and a comparison of CK-BB concentrations to prostate acid phosphatase concentration. J Nat Cancer Inst 1981; 66:659-662